First Edition

MEDICAL MANAGEMENT OF RADIOLOGICAL CASUALTIES

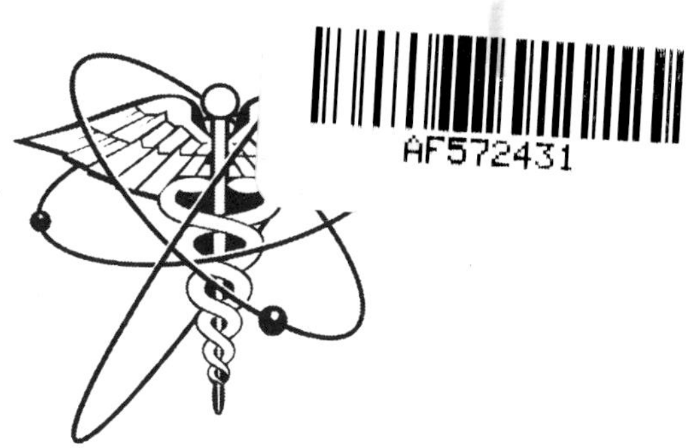

HANDBOOK

Military Medical Operations Office
Armed Forces Radiobiology Research Institute
Bethesda, Maryland 20889–5603
http://www.afrri.usuhs.mil

December 1999

First Edition

MEDICAL MANAGEMENT OF RADIOLOGICAL CASUALTIES

HANDBOOK

December 1999

Colonel David G. Jarrett

Medical Corps, United States Army

Comments and suggestions are solicited.
They should be addressed to:

Military Medical Operations
DSN 295-0316
meir@mx.afrri.usuhs.mil

Armed Forces Radiobiology Research Institute
8901 Wisconsin Avenue
Bethesda, MD 20889–5603

AFRRI Special Publication 99–2
Printed December 1999

This publication is a product of the Armed Forces Radiobiology Research Institute's Information Services Division. For more information about AFRRI publications, visit our Internet Web site at www.afrri.usuhs.mil or telephone 301–295–3536 or write AFRRI, 8901 Wisconsin Avenue, Bethesda, MD 20889–5603.

DISCLAIMER

The purpose of this handbook is to provide concise supplemental reading material for the Medical Effects of Ionizing Radiation Course, which is the only course in the Department of Defense for training health care professionals in the management of uncontrolled ionizing radiation exposure.

Mention of specific commercial equipment or therapeutic agents does not constitute endorsement by the Defense Department; trade names are used only for clarity of purpose. No therapeutic agents or regimens have been approved by the federal Food and Drug Administration (FDA) for the specific treatment of ionizing radiation injury. Ethical constraints bar the human-efficacy research protocols necessary to obtain this certification. Therapeutic agents described here have been FDA-approved for other purposes unless otherwise specified. It is the responsibility of the licensed medical provider to decide how best to use available therapy in the best interests of the patient.

Every effort has been made to make this handbook consistent with official policy and doctrine. However, the information contained in this handbook is not official Defense Department policy or doctrine, and it should not be construed as such unless it is supported by other documents.

ACKNOWLEDGMENTS

This handbook would not be possible without the assistance and support of Army Colonel Robert Eng, Dr. John Ainsworth, Navy Captain James Malinoski, Air Force Colonel Glenn Reeves, Navy Captain Steven Torrey, Air Force Colonel Curtis Pearson, Army Lieutenant Colonel Carl Curling, Air Force Lieutenant Colonel Richard Lofts, Army Lieutenant Colonel Charles Salter, Air Force Lieutenant Colonel Ming Chiang, Army Lieutenant Colonel Ross Pastel, Navy Lieutenant Commander Tyrone Naquin, Army Major Sharon Barnes, Navy Lieutenant Theodore St. John, Navy Lieutenant Bruce Holland, Navy Lieutenant Gregory Kahles, Army Captain Gerard Vavrina, Navy Lieutenant Rebecca Sine, Army Captain Christopher Pitcher, Dr. G. David Ledney, Dr. David Livengood, Dr. Terry Pellmar, Dr. William Blakely, Dr. Gregory Knudson, Dr. David McClain, Dr. Thomas Seed, Donna Solyan, Mark Behme, Carolyn Wooden, Guy Bateman, Jane Myers, and others too numerous to mention. The exclusion of anyone on this page is purely accidental and in no way lessens the gratitude we feel for contributions made to the Medical Radiological Defense Program of the United States of America and particularly this handbook.

Introduction

Nuclear Detonation and Other High-Dose Radiation Situations

Radiation Dispersal Device and Industrial Contamination Situations

Operational Aspects

Appendices

Contents

Tables

INTRODUCTION

Medical defense against radiological warfare is one of the least emphasized segments of modern medical education. Forty years of nuclear-doomsday predictions made any realistic preparation for radiation casualty management an untenable political consideration. The end of the Cold War has dramatically reduced the likelihood of strategic nuclear weapons use and thermonuclear war.

Unfortunately, the proliferation of nuclear material and technology has made the acquisition and adversarial use of ionizing radiation weapons more probable than ever. In the modern era, military personnel and their nation's population will expect that a full range of medical modalities will be employed to decrease the morbidity and mortality from the use of these weapons. Fortunately, treatment of radiation casualties is both effective and practical.

Prior to 1945, ionizing radiation was deemed nearly innocuous and often believed to be beneficial. Individual exposures to low-level radiation commonly occurred from cosmetics, luminous paints, medical-dental x-ray machines, and shoe-fitting apparatus in retail stores. The physical destruction caused by the nuclear explosions above Hiroshima and Nagasaki and the Civil Defense programs of the 1960's changed that perception.

Since that time, popular conceptions and misconceptions have permeated both attitudes and political doctrine. The significant radiological accidents at Chernobyl and Goiânia are models for the use of radiological weapons. To date, radiological warfare has been limited to demonstration events such as those by the Chechens in Moscow and threats by certain deposed third-world leaders.

As U.S. forces deploy to areas devastated by civil war and factional strife, unmarked radioactive material will be encountered in waste dumps, factories, abandoned medical clinics, and nuclear fuel facilities. Medical providers must be prepared to adequately treat injuries complicated by ionizing radiation exposure and radioactive contamination. To that end, the theory and treatment of radiological casualties is taught in the Medical Effects of Ionizing Radiation Course offered by the Armed Forces Radiobiology Research Institute at Bethesda, Maryland.

Radiation Threat Scenarios

A radiation dispersal device (RDD) is any device that causes the purposeful dissemination of radioactive material across an area without a nuclear detonation. Such a weapon can be easily developed and used by any combatant with conventional weapons and access to radionuclides. The material dispersed can originate from any location that uses radioactive sources, such as a nuclear waste processor, a nuclear power plant, a university research facility, a medical radiotherapy clinic, or an industrial complex. The radioactive source is blown up using conventional explosives and is scattered across the targeted area as debris.

This type of weapon would cause conventional casualties to become contaminated with radionuclides and would complicate medical evacuation within the contaminated area. It would function as either a terror weapon or terrain-denial mechanism. Many materials used in military ordnance, equipment, and supplies contain radioactive components. U.S. forces may be operating in a theater that has nuclear reactors that were not designed to U.S. specifications and are without containment vessels. These reactors may be lucrative enemy artillery or bombing targets.

Significant amounts of radioactive material may be deposited on surfaces after the use of any nuclear weapon or RDD, destruction of a nuclear reactor, a nuclear accident, or improper nuclear waste disposal. Military operations in these contaminated areas could result in military personnel receiving sufficient radiation exposure or particulate contamination to warrant medical evaluation and remediation.

Depleted uranium munitions on the battlefield do not cause a significant radiation hazard, although if vaporized and inhaled, they do pose the risk of heavy-metal toxicity to the kidneys. Materials such as industrial radiography units, damaged medical radiotherapy units, and old reactor fuel rods can be responsible for significant local radiation hazards.

Many nations may soon have the capability of constructing nuclear weapons. The primary limitation is the availability of weapons-grade fuel. Combatants with a limited stockpile of nuclear weapons or the capability of constructing improvised nuclear devices might use them either as desperation measures or for shock value against troop concentrations, political targets, or centers of mass. Small-yield tactical nuclear weapons might also be used in special situations.

Nuclear weapons might also be employed as a response to either the use or threat of use of any weapon of mass destruction. Large numbers of casualties with combined injuries would be generated from the periphery of the immediately lethal zone. Advanced medical care would be available outside the area of immediate destruction; consequently, primary management importance would be placed on evacuating casualties to a multiplicity of available medical centers throughout the United States.

Types of Ionizing Radiation

Alpha particles are massive, charged particles (4 times the mass of a neutron). Because of their size, alpha particles cannot travel far and are fully stopped by the dead layers of the skin or by a uniform. Alpha particles are a negligible external hazard, but when they are emitted from an internalized radionuclide source, they can cause significant cellular damage in the region immediately adjacent to their physical location.

Beta particles are very light, charged particles that are found primarily in fallout radiation. These particles can travel a short distance in tissue; if large quantities are involved, they can produce damage to the basal stratum of the skin. The lesion produced, a "beta burn," can appear similar to a thermal burn.

Gamma rays, emitted during a nuclear detonation and in fallout, are uncharged radiation similar to x rays. They are highly energetic and pass through matter easily. Because of its high penetrability, gamma radiation can result in whole-body exposure.

Neutrons, like gamma rays, are uncharged, are only emitted during the nuclear detonation, and are not a fallout hazard. However, neutrons have significant mass and interact with the nuclei of atoms, severely disrupting atomic structures. Compared to gamma rays, they can cause 20 times more damage to tissue.

When radiation interacts with atoms, energy is deposited, resulting in ionization (electron excitation). This ionization may damage certain critical molecules or structures in a cell. Two modes of action in the cell are direct and indirect action. The radiation may directly hit a particularly sensitive atom or molecule in the cell. The damage from this is irreparable; the cell either dies or is caused to malfunction.

The radiation can also damage a cell indirectly by interacting with water molecules in the body. The energy deposited in the water leads to the creation of unstable, toxic hyperoxide molecules; these then damage sensitive molecules and afflict subcellular structures.

Units of Radiation

The *radiation absorbed dose* (rad) is a measure of the energy deposited in matter by ionizing radiation. This terminology is being replaced by the International System skin dose unit for radiation absorbed dose, the gray (Gy) (1 joule per kilogram); 1 Gy = 100 rad; 10 milligray (mGy) = 1 rad. The dose in gray is a measure of absorbed dose in any material. The unit for dose, gray, is not restricted to any specific radiation, but can be used for all forms of ionizing radiation. Dose means the total amount of energy absorbed per gram of tissue. The exposure could be single or multiple and either short or long in duration.

Dose rate is the dose of radiation per unit of time.

Free-in-air dose refers to the radiation measured in air at a certain point. Free-in-air dose is exceedingly easy to measure with current field instruments, and more meaningful doses, such as midline tissue dose or dose to the blood-forming organs, may be estimated by approximation. Military tactical dosimeters measure free-in-air doses.

Different radiation types have more effects as their energy is absorbed in tissue. This difference is adjusted by use of a quality factor (QF). The dose in rads times the QF yields the rem, or *radiation equivalent, man*. The international unit for this radiation equivalency is the sievert (Sv) and is appropriately utilized when estimating long-term risks of radiation injury. Since the QF for x-ray or gamma radiation = 1, then for pure gamma radiation:

100 rad = 100 cGy = 1000 mGy = 1 Gy = 1 Sv = 100 rem

NUCLEAR DETONATION AND OTHER HIGH-DOSE RADIATION SITUATIONS

ACUTE HIGH-DOSE RADIATION

Acute high-dose radiation occurs in three principal tactical situations:

- A nuclear detonation will result in extremely high dose rates from radiation during the initial 60 seconds (prompt radiation) and then from the fission products present in the fallout area relatively close to ground zero.

- A second situation would occur when high-grade nuclear material is allowed to form a critical mass ("criticality"). The subsequent nuclear reaction then releases large amounts of gamma and neutron radiation without a nuclear explosion.

- A radiation dispersal device made from highly radioactive material such as cobalt-60 could also produce a dose high enough to cause acute injury.

The two most significant radiosensitive organ systems in the body are the hematopoietic and the gastrointestinal

(GI) systems. The relative sensitivity of an organ to direct radiation injury depends upon its component tissue sensitivities. Cellular effects of radiation, whether due to direct or indirect damage, are basically the same for the different kinds and doses of radiation.

The simplest effect is cell death. With this effect, the cell is no longer present to reproduce and perform its primary function.

Changes in cellular function can occur at lower radiation doses than those that cause cell death. Changes can include delays in phases of the mitotic cycle, disrupted cell growth, permeability changes, and changes in motility. In general, actively dividing cells are most sensitive to radiation. Radiosensitivity also tends to vary inversely with the degree of differentiation of the cell.

The severe radiation sickness resulting from external irradiation and its consequent organ effects is a primary medical concern. When appropriate medical care is *not* provided, the median lethal dose of radiation, the $LD_{50/60}$ (that which will kill 50% of the exposed persons within a period of 60 days), is estimated to be 3.5 Gy.

Recovery of a particular cell system is possible if a sufficient fraction of a given stem cell population remains after radiation injury. Although complete recovery may appear to occur, late somatic effects may have a higher probability of occurrence because of the radiation damage.

Modern medical care dramatically improves the survivability of radiation injury. Nearly all radiation casualties have a treatable injury if medical care can be made available to them. Casualties with unsurvivable irradiation are usually immediately killed or severely injured by the blast and thermal effects of a detonation. Unfortunately, significant doses of radiation below the level necessary to cause symptoms alter the body's immune response and sensitize the person to the effects of both biological and chemical weapons.

Effect on Bone-Marrow Cell Kinetics

The bone marrow contains three cell renewal systems: the erythropoietic (red cell), the myelopoietic (white cell), and the thrombopoietic (platelet). A single stem cell type gives rise to these three cell lines in the bone marrow, but their time cycles, cellular distribution patterns, and post-irradiation responses are quite different.

The erythropoietic system is responsible for the production of mature erythrocytes (red cells). This system has a marked propensity for regeneration following irradiation. After sublethal exposures, marrow erythropoiesis normally recovers slightly earlier than myelopoiesis and thrombopoiesis and occasionally overshoots the baseline level before levels at or near normal are reached. Reticulocytosis is occasionally evident in peripheral blood smears during the early intense regenerative phase occurring after maximum depression and often closely follows the temporal pattern of marrow erythropoietic recovery. Although anemia may be evident in the later stages of the bone-marrow syndrome, it should not be considered a survival-limiting factor.

The function of the myelopoietic cell renewal system is mainly to produce mature granulocytes, that is, neutrophils, eosinophils, and basophils, for the circulating blood. Neutrophils are the most important cell type in this cell line because of their role in combating infection. The most radiosensitive of these cells are the rapidly proliferating ones. The mature circulating neutrophil normally requires 3 to 7 days to form from its stem cell precursor stage in the bone marrow.

Mature granulocytes are available upon demand from venous, splenic, and bone-marrow pools. These pools are normally depleted soon after radiation-induced bone-marrow injury. Because of the rapid turnover in the granulocyte cell renewal system (approximately 8-day cellular life cycle), evidence of radiation damage to marrow myelopoiesis occurs in the peripheral blood within 2 to 4 days after whole-body irradiation.

Recovery of myelopoiesis lags slightly behind erythropoiesis and is accompanied by rapid increases in numbers of differentiating and dividing forms in the marrow. Prompt recovery is occasionally manifested and is indicated by increased numbers of band cells in the peripheral blood.

Platelets are produced by megakaryocytes in the bone marrow. Both platelets and mature megakaryocytes are relatively radioresistant; however, the stem cells and immature stages are very radiosensitive. The transit time through the megakaryocyte proliferating compartment in man ranges from 4 to 10 days. Platelets have a lifespan of 8 to 9 days. Platelet depression is influenced by the normal turnover kinetics of cells within the maturing and functional compartments.

Thrombocytopenia is reached by 3 to 4 weeks after midlethal-range doses and occurs from the killing of stem cells and immature megakaryocyte stages, with subsequent maturational depletion of functional megakaryocytes. Regeneration of thrombocytopoiesis after sublethal irradiation normally lags behind both erythropoiesis and myelopoiesis.

Supranormal platelet numbers overshooting the preirradiation level have occurred during the intense regenerative phase in human nuclear accident victims. Blood coagulation defects with concomitant hemorrhage constitute important clinical sequelae during the thrombocytopenic phase of bone-marrow and gastrointestinal syndromes.

Gastrointestinal Kinetics

The vulnerability of the small intestine to radiation is primarily in the cell renewal system of the intestinal villi. Epithelial cell formation, migration, and loss occur in the crypt and villus structures. Stem cells and proliferating cells move from crypts into the necks of the crypts and bases of the villi. Functionally mature epithelial cells migrate up the villus wall and are extruded at the villus tip.

The overall transit time from stem cell to extrusion on the villus for humans is estimated as being 7 to 8 days.

Because of the high turnover rate occurring within the stem cell and proliferating cell compartment of the crypt, marked damage occurs in this region from whole-body radiation doses above the midlethal range. Destruction as well as mitotic inhibition occur within the highly radiosensitive crypt cells within hours after high doses. Maturing and functional epithelial cells continue to migrate up the villus wall and are extruded, albeit the process is slowed. Shrinkage of villi and morphological changes in mucosal cells occur as new cell production is diminished within the crypts.

Continued loss of epithelial cells in the absence of cell production results in denudation of the intestinal mucosa. Concomitant injury to the microvasculature of the mucosa results in hemorrhage and marked fluid and electrolyte loss contributing to shock. These events normally occur within 1 to 2 weeks after irradiation.

Radiation-Induced Early Transient Incapacitation

Early transient incapacitation (ETI) is associated with very high acute doses of radiation. In humans, it has only occurred during fuel reprocessing accidents. The lower limit is probably 20 to 40 Gy. The latent period, a return of partial functionality, is very short, varying from several hours to 1 to 3 days. Subsequently, a deteriorating state of consciousness with vascular instability and death is typical. Convulsions without increased intracranial pressure may or may not occur.

Personnel close enough to a nuclear explosion to develop ETI would die due to blast and thermal effects. However, in nuclear detonations above the atmosphere with essentially no blast, very high fluxes of ionizing radiation may extend out far enough to result in high radiation doses to aircraft crews. Such personnel could conceivably manifest this syndrome, uncomplicated by blast or thermal injury. Also, personnel protected from blast and thermal effects in shielded areas could also sustain such doses. Doses in this range could also result from military operations in a reactor facility or fuel reprocessing plant where personnel are accidentally or deliberately wounded by a nuclear criticality event.

Time Profile

Acute radiation syndrome (ARS) is a sequence of phased symptoms. Symptoms vary with individual radiation sensitivity, type of radiation, and the radiation dose absorbed. The extent of symptoms will heighten and the duration of each phase will shorten with increasing radiation dose.

Prodromal Phase

The prodrome is characterized by the relatively rapid onset of nausea, vomiting, and malaise. This is a nonspecific clinical response to acute radiation exposure. An early onset of symptoms in the absence of associated trauma suggests a large radiation exposure. Radiogenic vomiting may easily be confused with psychogenic vomiting that often results from stress and realistic fear reactions. Use of oral prophylactic antiemetics, such as granisetron (Kytril®) and ondansetron (Zofran®), may be indicated in situations where high-dose radiological exposure is likely or unavoidable. The purpose of the drug would be to reduce other traumatic injuries after irradiation by maintaining short-term full physical capability.

These medications will diminish the nausea and vomiting in a significant percentage of those personnel exposed and consequently decrease the likelihood of a compromised individual being injured because he was temporarily debilitated. The prophylactic antiemetics do not change the degree of injury due to irradiation and are not radioprotectants. They do diminish the reliability of nausea and emesis as indicators of radiation exposure.

Latent Period

Following recovery from the prodromal phase, the exposed individual will be relatively symptom free. The length of this phase varies with the dose. The latent phase is longest preceding the bone-marrow depression of the hematopoietic syndrome and may vary between 2 and 6 weeks.

The latent period is somewhat shorter prior to the gastrointestinal syndrome, lasting from a few days to a week.

It is shortest of all preceding the neurovascular syndrome, lasting only a matter of hours. These times are exceedingly variable and may be modified by the presence of other disease or injury. Because of the extreme variability, it is not practical to hospitalize all personnel suspected of having radiation injury early in the latent phase.

Manifest Illness

This phase presents with the clinical symptoms associated with the major organ system injured (marrow, intestinal, neurovascular). A summary of essential features of each syndrome and the doses at which they would be seen in young healthy adults exposed to short, high-dose single exposures is shown in appendix C. The details of the clinical courses of each of the three syndromes are also described.

Clinical Acute Radiation Syndrome

Patients who have received doses of radiation between 0.7 and 4 Gy will have depression of bone-marrow function leading to pancytopenia. Changes within the peripheral blood profile will occur as early as 24 hours post-irradiation. Lymphocytes will be depressed most rapidly; other leukocytes and thrombocytes will be depressed somewhat less rapidly.

Decreased resistance to infection and anemia will vary considerably from as early as 10 days to as much as 6 to 8 weeks after exposure. Erythrocytes are least affected due to their useful lifespan in circulation.

The average time of onset of clinical problems of bleeding and anemia and decreased resistance to infection is 2 to 3 weeks. Even potentially lethal cases of bone-marrow depression may not occur until 6 weeks after exposure. The presence of other injuries will increase the severity and accelerate the time of maximum bone-marrow depression.

The most useful forward laboratory procedure to evaluate marrow depression is the peripheral blood count. A 50% drop in lymphocytes within 24 hours indicates significant radiation injury. Bone-marrow studies will rarely be possible under field conditions and will add little information to that which can be obtained from a careful peripheral blood count. Early therapy should prevent nearly all deaths from marrow injury alone.

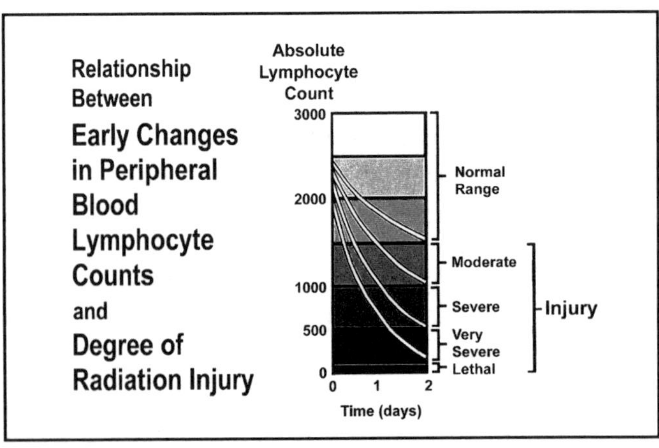

Higher single gamma-ray doses of radiation (6–8 Gy) will result in the gastrointestinal syndrome, and it will almost always be accompanied by bone-marrow suppression. After a short latent period of a few days to a week or so, the characteristic severe fluid losses, hemorrhage, and diarrhea begin. Derangement of the luminal epithelium and injury to the fine vasculature of the submucosa lead to loss of intestinal mucosa. Peripheral blood counts done on these patients will show the early onset of a severe pancytopenia occurring as a result of bone-marrow depression. Radiation enteropathy consequently does not result in an inflammatory response.

It must be assumed during the care of all patients that even those with a typical gastrointestinal syndrome may be salvageable. Replacement of fluids and prevention of infection by bacterial transmigration is mandatory.

The neurovascular syndrome is associated only with very high acute doses of radiation (20–40 Gy). Hypotension may be seen at lower doses. The latent period is very short, varying from several hours to 1 to 3 days. The clinical picture is of a steadily deteriorating state of consciousness with eventual coma and death. Convulsions may or may not occur, and there may be little or no indication of increased intracranial pressure. Because of the very high doses of radiation required to cause this syndrome, personnel close enough to a nuclear explosion to receive such high doses would generally be located well within the range of 100% lethality due to blast and thermal effects.

Doses in this range could also result from military

operations in a reactor facility or fuel reprocessing plant where personnel are accidentally or deliberately exposed to a nuclear criticality event. Still, very few patients will be hospitalized with this syndrome, and it is the only category of radiation injury where the triage classification "expectant" is appropriate.

Chemical Weapons and Radiation

Mustard agents and radiation can cause many similar effects at the cellular level. Their use in combination will have a geometric effect on morbidity. Research into these effects is only just beginning. The immediate effects of the chemical agents must be countered before attention is paid to the effects of radiation, which may not manifest for days or weeks.

Little is known about the combined effect of radiation and nerve agents. Radiation will lower the threshold for seizure activity and may potentiate the effects on the central nervous system.

Biological Weapons and Radiation

The primary cause of death from radiation injury is infection by normal pathogens during the phase of manifest illness. Even minimally symptomatic doses of radiation depress the immune response and will dramatically increase the infectivity and apparent virulence of biological agents. Biological weapons may be significantly more devastating against an irradiated population. Early research with radiation injury and an anthrax simulant demonstrates that significantly fewer spores are required to induce infection. Computer simulations using these parameter changes yield orders of magnitude increases in casualties. Usually ineffective portals of infection that are made accessible by partial immunoincompetence may cause unusual infection profiles.

Immunization efficacy will be diminished if instituted prior to complete immune system recovery. Use of live-agent vaccines after irradiation injury could conceivably result in disseminated infection with the inoculation strain. There are currently insufficient data to reliably predict casualties from combined injuries of subclinical or sublethal doses of ionizing radiation and exposure to aerosols with a biological warfare agent. Research suggests a shortened fatal course of disease when virulent-strain virus is injected into sublethally irradiated test models.

MANAGEMENT PROTOCOL FOR ACUTE RADIATION SYNDROME

The medical management of radiation and combined injuries can be divided into three stages: triage, emergency care, and definitive care. During triage, patients are prioritized and rendered immediate lifesaving care. Emergency care includes therapeutics and diagnostics necessary during the first 12 to 24 hours. Definitive care is rendered when final disposition and therapeutic regimens are established.

Effective quality care can be provided both when there are few casualties and a well-equipped facility and when there are many casualties and a functioning worldwide evacuation system. The therapeutic modalities will vary according to current medical knowledge and experience, the number of casualties, available medical facilities, and resources. Recommendations for the treatment of a few casualties may not apply to the treatment of mass casualties because of limited resources. A primary goal should be the evacuation of a radiation casualty prior to the onset of manifest illness.

Prodromal symptoms begin within hours of exposure. They include nausea, vomiting, diarrhea, fatigue, weakness, fever, and headache. The prodromal gastrointestinal symptoms generally do not last longer than 24 to 48 hours after exposure, but a vague weakness and fatigue can persist for an undetermined length of time. The time of onset, severity, and duration of these signs are dose dependent and dose-rate dependent. They can be used in conjunction with white blood cell differential counts to determine the presence and severity of the acute radiation syndrome.

Both the rate and degree of decrease in blood cells are dose dependent. A useful rule of thumb: If lymphocytes have decreased by 50% and are less than 1 x 10^9/l (1000/μl) within 24 to 48 hours, the patient has received at least a moderate dose of radiation. In combined injuries, lymphocytes may be an unreliable indicator. Patients with severe burns and/or trauma to more than one system often develop lymphopenia. These injuries should be assessed by standard procedures, keeping in mind that the signs and symptoms of tissue injuries can mimic and obscure those caused by acute radiation effects.

Conventional Therapy for Neutropenia and Infection

The prevention and management of infection is the mainstay of therapy. Antibiotic prophylaxis should only be considered in afebrile patients at the highest risk for infection. These patients have profound neutropenia (< 0.1 x 10^9 cells/l (100 cells/μl)) that has an expected duration of greater than 7 days. The degree of neutropenia (absolute neutrophil count [ANC] < 100/μl) is the greatest risk factor for developing infection. As the duration of neutropenia increases, the risk of secondary infections such as invasive mycoses also increases. For these reasons, adjuvant therapies such as the use of cytokines will prove invaluable in the treatment of the severely irradiated person.

Prevention of Infection

Initial care of medical casualties with moderate and severe radiation exposure should probably include early institution of measures to reduce pathogen acquisition, with emphasis on low-microbial-content food, acceptable water supplies, frequent hand washing (or wearing of gloves), and air filtration. During the neutropenic period, prophylactic use of selective gut decontamination with

> **Basic Principles**
>
> *Principle 1*: The spectrum of infecting organisms and antimicrobial susceptibility patterns vary both among institutions and over time.
>
> *Principle 2*: Life-threatening, gram-negative bacterial infections are universal among neutropenic patients, but the prevalence of life-threatening, gram-positive bacterial infections varies greatly among institutions.
>
> *Principle 3*: Current empiric antimicrobial regimens are highly effective for initial management of febrile, neutropenic episodes.
>
> *Principle 4*: The nidus of infection (i.e., the reason the patient is infected) must be identified and eliminated.

antibiotics that suppress aerobes but preserve anaerobes is recommended. The use of sucralfate or prostaglandin analogs may prevent gastric hemorrhage without decreasing gastric activity. When possible, early oral feeding is preferred to intravenous feeding to maintain the immunologic and physiologic integrity of the gut.

Overall Recommendations

1. A standardized plan for the management of febrile, neutropenic patients must be devised.
2. Empiric regimens must contain antibiotics broadly active against gram-negative bacteria, but antibiotics directed against gram-positive bacteria need be included only in institutions where these infections are prevalent.
3. No single antimicrobial regimen can be recommended above all others, as pathogens and susceptibility vary with time.
4. If infection is documented by cultures, the empiric regimen may require adjustment to provide appropriate coverage for the isolate. This should not narrow the antibiotic spectrum.
5. If the patient defervesces and remains afebrile, the initial regimen should be continued for a minimum of 7 days.

Management of Infection

The management of established or suspected infection (neutropenia and fever) in irradiated persons is similar to that used for other febrile neutropenic patients, such as solid tumor patients receiving chemotherapy. An empirical regimen of antibiotics should be selected, based on the pattern of bacterial susceptibility and nosocomial infections in the particular institution. Broad-spectrum empiric therapy with high doses of one or more antibiotics should be used, avoiding aminoglycosides whenever feasible due to associated toxicities. Therapy should be continued until the patient is afebrile for 24 hours and the ANC is greater than or equal to 0.5×10^9 cells/l (500 cells/μl). Combination regimens often prove to be more effective than monotherapy. The potential for additivity or synergy should be present in the choice of antibiotics.

Hematopoietic Growth Factors

Hematopoietic growth factors, such as filgrastim (Neupogen®), a granulocyte colony-stimulating factor (G–CSF), and sargramostim (Leukine®), a granulocyte-macrophage colony-stimulating factor (GM–CSF), are potent stimulators of hematopoiesis and shorten the time to recovery of neutrophils (table 1). The risk of infection and subsequent complications are directly related to depth and duration of neutropenia.

Clinical support should be in the form of antibiotics and fresh, irradiated platelets and blood products. Used concurrently with filgrastim or sargramostim, a marked reduction in infectious complications translates to reduced morbidity and mortality. The longer the duration of severe neutropenia, the greater the risk of secondary infections. An additional benefit of the CSFs is their ability to increase the functional capacity of the neutrophil and thereby contribute to the prevention of infection as an active part of cellular host defense.

Table 1. Recommendations for use of cytokines for patients expected to experience severe neutropenia.

Filgrastim (G–CSF)	2.5–5 μg/kg/d QD s.c. (100–200 $\mu g/m^2/d$)
Sargramostim (GM–CSF)	5–10 μg/kg/d QD s.c. (200–400 $\mu g/m^2/d$)

In order to achieve maximum clinical response, filgrastim or sargramostim should be started 24 to 72 hours subsequent to the exposure. This provides the opportunity for maximum recovery. Cytokine administration should continue, with consecutive daily injections, to reach the desired effect of an ANC of 10 x 10^9/l.

BLAST AND THERMAL BIOLOGICAL EFFECTS

The blast and thermal biological effects of nuclear weapons are caused by the explosive forces generated. The physically most destructive forces are pressures and winds, the thermal pulse, and secondary fires. Psychological effects include intense acute and chronic stress disorders. Fallout and radiation dispersal devices may have limited acute effects but can have significant long-term effects.

Blast Injury

Two basic types of blast forces occur simultaneously in a nuclear detonation blast wave. They are direct blast wave overpressure forces and indirect blast wind drag forces.

Blast wind drag forces are the most important medical casualty-producing effects. Direct overpressure effects do not extend out as far from the point of detonation and are frequently masked by drag force effects as well as by thermal effects.

The drag forces are proportional to the velocities and durations of the winds, which in turn vary with distance from the point of detonation, yield of the weapon, and altitude of the burst. These winds are relatively short in duration but are extremely severe. They can be much greater in velocity than the strongest hurricane winds. Considerable injury can result, due either to missiles (table 2) or to casualties being blown against objects and structures in the environment (translational injuries).

Personnel in fortifications or armored vehicles who are protected from thermal and blast wind may be subjected to complex patterns of direct overpressures, since blast waves can enter such structures and be reflected and reinforced within them. Important variables of the blast wave include the rate of pressure rise at the blast wave front, the magnitude of the peak overpressure, and the duration of the blast wave.

Blast casualties will require evaluation for acute trauma in accordance with advanced trauma life-support

Table 2. Probabilities of serious injury from small missiles.

	Range (km) for probability of		
Yield (kt)	1%	50%	99%
1	0.28	0.22	0.17
10	0.73	0.57	0.44
20	0.98	0.76	0.58
50	1.4	1.1	0.84
100	1.9	1.5	1.1
200	2.5	1.9	1.5
500	3.6	2.7	2.1
1000	4.8	3.6	2.7

standard therapies. Pneumothorax secondary to both direct and indirect trauma and pneumoperitoneum can be treated by appropriate surgical intervention. Subsequent delayed sequelae such as pulmonary failure may result from severe barotrauma.

Response to therapy will be complicated by immune system compromise and delayed wound healing due to any concomitant irradiation. Open wounds will require thorough debridement and removal of all contaminants, including radioactive debris. Suspected fractures should be splinted. Spinal injuries resulting from either translational injury or blunt force trauma should be treated with immobilization.

In the presence of traumatic injury, hypotension must be considered to be due to hypovolemia and not to concomitant head or radiological injury. Surgical priorities for acute or life-threatening injury must precede any treatment priority for associated radiation injury. Treatment of tympanic membrane rupture can be delayed.

The drag forces of the blast winds are strong enough to displace even large objects such as vehicles or to cause buildings to collapse. These events will result in serious crush injuries, comparable to those seen in earthquakes and bombings. When the human body is hurled against fixed objects, the probability and the severity of injury are functions of the velocity of the body at the time of impact. Table 3 shows terminal or impact velocities associated with significant but nonlethal blunt injury.

Table 3. Ranges for selected impact velocities of a 70-kg human body displaced 3 m by blast wind drag forces.

Weapon yield (kt)	Range (km) for velocities (m/sec) of		
	2.6	6.6	17.0
1	0.38	0.27	0.19
10	1.0	0.75	0.53
20	1.3	0.99	0.71
50	1.9	1.4	1.0
100	2.5	1.9	1.4
200	3.2	2.5	1.9
500	4.6	3.6	2.7
1000	5.9	4.8	3.6

Wounds and Radiation

Wounds that are left open and allowed to heal by secondary intention will serve as a potentially fatal nidus of infection in the radiologically injured patient. Wound healing is markedly compromised within hours of radiation injury. If at all possible, wounds should be closed primarily as soon as possible. Extensive debridement of wounds may be necessary in order to allow this closure.

Traditionally, combat wounds are not closed primarily due to the high level of contamination, devitalized tissue, and the subsequent morbidity and mortality of the closed-space contamination. In the case of the radiation/

combined injury patient, aggressive therapy will be required to allow survival.

The decision to amputate an extremity that in ordinary circumstances would be salvageable will rest with the surgeon in the first 2 days following the combined injury. No studies are available regarding the use of aggressive marrow resuscitation as described for the physically wounded patient.

All surgical procedures must be accomplished within 36 to 48 hours of radiation injury. If surgery cannot be completed at far-forward locations, patients with moderate injury will need early evacuation to a level where surgical facilities are immediately available.

Thermal Injuries

Thermal burns will be the most common injuries, subsequent to both the thermal pulse and the fires it ignites. The thermal radiation emitted by a nuclear detonation causes burns in two ways, by direct absorption of the thermal energy through exposed surfaces (flash burns) or by the indirect action of fires caused in the environment (flame burns).

Since the thermal pulse is direct infrared, burn patterns will be dictated by location and clothing pattern. Exposed skin will absorb the infrared, and the victim will be burned on the side facing the explosion. Light colors will reflect the infrared, while dark portions of clothing will absorb it and cause pattern burns. Skin shaded from the direct light of the blast will be protected. Any object between personnel and the fireball will provide a measure of protection, but close to the fireball, the thermal output is so great that everything is incinerated. Obviously, immediate lethality would be 100% within this range. The actual range out to which overall lethality would be 100% will vary with yield, position of burst, weather, and the environment.

Protection from burns can be achieved with clothing. That protection, however, is not absolute. The amount of heat energy conducted across clothing is a function of the energy absorbed by and the thermal conducting properties of the clothing. Loose, light-colored clothing significantly reduces the effective range, producing partial thickness burns, thus affording significant protection against thermal flash burns.

Firestorm and secondary fires will cause typical flame burns, but they will be compounded by closed-space fire-associated injuries. Patients with toxic gas injury from burning plastics and other material, superheated air inhalation burns, steam burns from ruptured pipes, and all other large conflagration-type injuries will present for treatment.

Indirect or flame burns result from exposure to fires caused by the thermal effects in the environment. Complications arise in the treatment of skin burns created, in part, from melting of manmade fibers. Clothing made of natural fibers should be worn next to the skin. The burns themselves will be far less uniform in degree and will not be limited to exposed surfaces. For example, the respiratory system may be exposed to the effects of hot gases. Respiratory system burns are associated with severe morbidity and high mortality rates. Early endotracheal intubation is advisable whenever airway burns are suspected.

Burns and Radiation

Mortality of thermal burns markedly increases with irradiation. Burns with 50% mortality may be transformed into 90+% mortality by concomitant radiation doses as small as 1.5 Gy. Aggressive marrow resuscitative therapeutic protocols may diminish this effect. Infection is the primary cause of death in these patients. Surgeons must decide early as to appropriate individual wound management. Full-thickness burns are ideal bacterial culture media, and excision of these burns may be indicated to allow primary closure. No changes should be made in the indications for escharotomy.

No studies are available regarding the use of modern skin graft techniques in irradiation injury victims. Use of topical antimicrobials whose side-effects include leukopenia may be a complicating factor in radiation-immunocompromised patients. No data are available regarding the response to clostridial infection, and strong consideration should be given to the use of passive tetanus immunization even in previously immunized patients.

Patients whose burns are contaminated by radioactive material should be gently decontaminated to minimize absorption through the burned skin. Most radiological contaminants will remain in the burn eschar when it sloughs.

Eye Injuries

The sudden exposures to high-intensity visible light and infrared radiation of a detonation will cause eye injury specifically to the chorioretinal areas. Optical equipment such as binoculars will increase the likelihood of damage. Eye injury is due not only to infrared energy but also to photochemical reactions that occur within the retina with light wavelengths in the range of 400 to 500 μm.

Those individuals looking directly at the flash will receive retinal burns. Night vision apparatus (NVA) electronically amplifies and reproduces the visual display. The NVA does not amplify the infrared and damaging wavelengths and will not cause retinal injury.

Flashblindness occurs with peripheral observation of a brilliant flash of intense light energy, for example, a fireball. This is a temporary condition that results from a depletion of photopigment from the retinal receptors. The duration of flash blindness can last several seconds when the exposure occurs during daylight. The blindness will then be followed by a darkened afterimage that lasts for several minutes. At night, flash blindness can last for up to 30 minutes.

RADIATION DISPERSAL DEVICE AND INDUSTRIAL CONTAMINATION SITUATIONS

LOW DOSE-RATE RADIATION

Late or delayed effects of radiation occur following a wide range of doses and dose rates. Delayed effects may appear months to years after irradiation and include a wide variety of effects involving almost all tissues or organs. Some of the possible delayed consequences of radiation injury are life shortening, carcinogenesis, cataract formation, chronic radiodermatitis, decreased fertility, and genetic mutations. The effect upon future generations is unclear. Data from Japan and Russia have not demonstrated significant genetic effects in humans.

Delivering the same gamma radiation dose at a much lower dose rate, or in fractions over a long period of time, allows tissue repair to occur. There is a consequent decrease in the total level of injury that would be expected from a single dose of the same magnitude delivered over a short period of time. Neutron-radiation damage does not appear to be dose-rate dependent.

Chronic Radiation Syndrome

When the Soviet Union developed its nuclear weapons program, safety procedures were often neglected to accelerate the production of plutonium. Workers were often exposed to radiation at annual doses of 2 to 4.5 Gy. The diagnosis of chronic radiation syndrome (CRS) was made in 1596 workers. CRS was defined as a complex clinical syndrome occurring as a result of the long-term exposure to single or total radiation doses that regularly exceed the permissible occupational dose. The clinical course was marked by neuroregulatory disorders, moderate to marked leukopenia (both neutrophils and lymphocytes depressed), and thrombocytopenia. In severe cases, anemia, atrophic changes in the gastrointestinal mucous membranes, encephalomyelitis, and infectious complications due to immune depression were noted.

CRS is highly unlikely to affect military personnel in operational settings. Prolonged deployments to heavily contaminated areas or long-term ingestion of highly contaminated food or water would be required. A near-ground weapon detonation, radiation dispersion device, major reactor accident, or similar event that creates contamination with high dose rates, given prolonged exposure, would permit development of this syndrome.

Persons who have been exposed to radiation for at least 3 years and have received at least 1 Gy or more to the marrow may develop CRS. It has only been described in the area of the former Soviet Union. Clinical symptoms are diffuse and may include sleep and/or appetite disturbances, generalized weakness and easy fatigability, increased excitability, loss of concentration, impaired memory, mood changes, vertigo, ataxia, paresthesias, headaches, epistaxis, chills, syncopal episodes, bone pain, and hot flashes.

Clinical findings may include localized bone or muscle tenderness, mild hypotension, tachycardia, intention tremor, ataxia, asthenia, hyperreflexia (occasionally hyporeflexia), delayed menarche, and underdeveloped secondary sexual characteristics. Laboratory findings include mild to marked pancytopenia and bone dysplasia. Gastric hypoacidity and dystrophic changes may be present. Once the patient is removed from the radiation environment, clinical symptoms and findings slowly resolve, and complete recovery has occurred from the lower doses.

Carcinogenesis

A stochastic effect is a consequence based on statistical probability. For radiation, tumor induction is the most important long-term sequelae for a dose of less than 1 Gy. Most of the data used to construct risk estimates are taken from radiation doses greater than 1 Gy and then extrapolated down for low-dose probability estimates. Significant direct data are not available for absolute risk determination of doses less than 100 mGy. In the case of the various radiation-induced cancers seen in humans, the latency period may be several years.

It is difficult to address the radiation-induced cancer risk of an individual person due to the already high background risk of developing cancer. Exposure to 100 mGy gamma radiation (2 times the U.S. occupational annual limit of 0.05 Gy) causes an 0.8% increase in lifetime risk of death from cancer. The general U.S. population has an annual lifetime risk for fatal cancer of 20%. If 5000 individuals are exposed to the notational 100-mGy level, then 40 additional people may eventually develop a fatal cancer. The fatal cancer incidences of 1000 in the group would increase to 1040 cases.

Cataract Formation

Deterministic effects are those that are directly dose related. While variations will occur due to individual sensitivity, the intensity of the effect is still directly dose related. Ocular cataract formation may begin anywhere from 6 months to several years after exposure. The threshold for detectable cataract formation is 2 Sv for acute gamma-radiation doses and 15 Sv for protracted doses. While all types of ionizing radiation may induce cataract formation, neutron irradiation is especially effective in its formation, even at relatively low doses.

Decreased Fertility

Despite the high degree of radiosensitivity of some stages of germ cell development, the testes and ovaries are only transiently affected by single sublethal doses of whole-body irradiation and generally go on to recover normal function. Whole-body irradiation above 120 mGy causes abrupt decreases in sperm count. A transient azoospermia will appear at sublethal radiation doses. The resulting sterility may last several months to several years, but recovery of natural fertility does occur.

When aberrations occur in germ cells, the effects may be reflected in subsequent generations. Most frequently, the aberrant stem cells do not produce mature sperm or ova, and no abnormalities are transmitted. If the abnormalities are not severe enough to prevent fertilization, the developing embryos will not be viable in most instances. Only when the chromosome damage is very slight and there is no actual loss of genetic material will the offspring be viable and abnormalities be transferable to succeeding generations.

These point mutations become important at low radiation dose levels. In any population of cells, spontaneous point mutations occur naturally. Radiation increases the rate of these mutations and thus potentially increases the abnormal genetic burden of future cellular generations.

This has not been documented in humans.

Fetal Exposure

The four main effects of ionizing radiation on the fetus are growth retardation; severe congenital malformations (including errors of metabolism); embryonic, fetal, or neonatal death; and carcinogenesis. Irradiation in the fetal period leads to the most pronounced permanent growth retardation.

The peak incidence of teratogenesis, or gross malformations, occurs when the fetus is irradiated during organogenesis. Radiation-induced malformations of bodily structures other than the central nervous system are uncommon in humans. Data on A-bomb survivors indicate that microcephaly may result from a free-in-air dose of 100 to 190 mGy.

Diagnostic x-ray irradiation at low doses *in utero* increases the cancer incidence by a factor of 1.5 to 2 during the first 10 to 15 years of life. It is assumed for practical purposes that the developing organism is susceptible to radiation-induced carcinogenesis. The maximum permissible dose to the fetus during gestation is 5 mSv, which treats the unborn child as a member of the general public brought involuntarily into controlled areas.

PSYCHOLOGICAL EFFECTS

Radiation illness symptoms in just a few soldiers can produce devastating psychological effects on an entire unit that is uninformed about the physical hazards of radiation. This acute anxiety has the potential to become the dominant source of cognitive stress in a unit. Soldiers are then more likely to focus on radiation detection and thus increase the potential of injury from conventional battlefield hazards.

Casualties should be treated with the primary combat psychology maxims of proximity, immediacy, and expectancy (P.I.E.) in order to minimize long-term casualties. Treat close to the unit, as early as possible, and communicate to them expectations that they will return to their units.

Nuclear Detonation

Devastation from a nuclear explosion will add to combat intensity and consequently increase stress casualties. The number of combat stress casualties depends on the leadership, cohesiveness, and morale of a unit. Positive combat stress behaviors such as altruism and loyalty to comrades will occur more frequently in units with exceptional *esprit de corps*.

Survivor guilt, anticipation of a lingering death, large physical casualty numbers, and delayed evacuation all contribute to acute stress. Radiation casualties deemed "expectant" due to severe neurological symptoms will add to this stress, particularly for medical professionals.

Radiation Dispersal Device (RDD)

The severity of the psychological effects of an RDD will depend on the nature of the RDD material itself and the method of deployment. A point source of radiation produces physical injury only to soldiers within its immediate vicinity. An RDD that uses a conventional explosion as a dispersal method will cause psychological injury from the physical effects of the blast in addition to the radiation and heavy-metal hazard inherent in many radioactive materials. Misinterpretation of the explosion as a nuclear detonation may induce psychological effects similar to those produced by a true nuclear detonation. The number of casualties from the blast and a generally more frantic situation will intensify the level of stress on soldiers.

The presence of an RDD within a civilian population center will produce more detrimental psychological damage to soldiers than would a military target. Military units in a theater of operation during war often have limited contact with civilian populations. However, during peacetime missions such as operations other than war (OOTW), a closer relationship may exist between civilians and soldiers. Treatment of civilian casualties, particularly children, from exposure to an RDD during an OOTW could markedly increase the psychological impact on soldiers.

Mass psychosomatic symptoms from the unrealistic fear of the effects of radioactive material pervasive in many civilian populations could severely overload both medical support and operations.

Contamination or Fallout Fields

An increase in combat stress is expected from the combined effects of chemical toxicity and radiation illness.

Lack of information and threat of exposure to radioactive material contribute to combat stress symptoms. Any activity in a potentially contaminated but unsurveilled area requires the use of MOPP (mission-oriented protective posture) gear, thus degrading unit performance. The difficulties in providing accurate definition of the boundaries of contamination are a significant source of anxiety. The amount of training as well as the intensity, duration, and degree of involvement will also contribute to combat stress. Prior identification of contamination is the most effective method of ensuring successful accomplishment of the unit mission.

The feeling of being under attack but not able to strike back and a lack of information will contribute to cognitive stress levels and the development of combat stress symptoms. The most extreme psychological damage occurs when physiological symptoms signal contact with chemical hazards. This type of "biodosimetry" will severely degrade the morale of the unit and confidence in a unit's leadership.

Long-term effects of toxicity cause soldiers to suffer from chronic psychological stress. This stress arises from uncertainty about one's ultimate fate as a result of exposure to radiation. The development of phobias, general depression and malaise, and posttraumatic stress disorder are possible. A variety of psychosomatic symptoms may arise as a result of acute anxiety about the effects of both toxicity and radiation.

EXTERNAL CONTAMINATION

External contamination by radionuclides will occur when a soldier traverses a contaminated area without appropriate barrier clothing. If the individual is wounded while in the contaminated area, he will become an externally contaminated patient. The radioactive-contamination hazard of injured personnel to both the patient and attending medical personnel will be negligible, so necessary medical or surgical treatment must not be delayed because of possible contamination. Unlike chemical contaminants, radiological material active enough to be an immediate threat can be detected at great distances.

Radiation detectors can locate external radioactive material. The most common contaminants will primarily emit alpha and beta radiation. Gamma-radiation emitters may cause whole-body irradiation. Beta emitters when left on the skin will cause significant burns and scarring. Alpha radiation does not penetrate the epithelium. It is impossible for a patient to be so contaminated that he is a radiation hazard to health care providers. External contamination of the skin and hair is particulate matter that can be washed off.

Chronic Radiodermatitis

Delayed, irreversible changes of the skin usually do not develop as a result of sublethal whole-body irradiation, but instead follow higher doses limited to the skin. These changes could occur with RDDs if there is heavy contamination of bare skin with beta-emitting materials. Beta-induced skin ulceration should be easily prevented with reasonable hygiene and would be particularly rare in climates where the soldiers were fully clothed (arms, legs, and neck covered). Table 4 lists the degrees of radiation dermatitis for local skin area radiation doses.

Table 4. Radiation dermatitis.

Radiation	Dose	Effect
	6–20 Sv	Erythema only
Acute	20–40 Sv	Skin breakdown in 2 wk
	> 3000 Sv	Immediate skin blistering
Chronic	> 20 Sv	Dermatitis, with cancer risk

Washing off the contaminants can prevent beta skin damage. If practical, the effluent should be sequestered and disposed of appropriately. Normal hospital barrier clothing is adequate to prevent contamination of medical personnel.

Decontamination

Decontamination is usually performed during the care of such patients by the emergency service and, ideally, prior to arrival at medical facilities. As this will not always be possible, decontamination procedures should be part of the operational plans and guides of all divisions and departments. This ensures flexibility of response and action and will prevent delay in needed medical treatment. The simple removal of outer clothing and shoes will, in most instances, effect a 90% reduction in the patient's contamination.

The presence of radiological contamination can be readily confirmed by passing a radiation detector (radiac) over the entire body. Open wounds should be covered prior to decontamination. Contaminated clothing should be carefully removed, placed in marked plastic bags, and removed to a secure location within a contaminated area. Bare skin and hair should be thoroughly washed, and if practical, the effluent should be sequestered and disposed of appropriately.

Radiological decontamination should never interfere with medical care. Unlike chemical agents, radioactive particles will not cause acute injury, and decontamination sufficient to remove chemical agents is more than sufficient to remove radiological contamination.

INTERNAL CONTAMINATION

Internal contamination will occur when unprotected personnel ingest, inhale, or are wounded by radioactive material. Any externally contaminated casualty who did not have respiratory protection should be evaluated for internal contamination. Metabolism of the nonradioactive analog determines the metabolic pathway of a radionuclide. Contamination evaluation and therapy must never take precedence over treatment of acute injury.

Distribution and Metabolism

The routes of intake are inhalation, ingestion, wound contamination, and skin absorption.

Within the respiratory tract, particles less than 5 microns in diameter may be deposited in the alveolar area. Larger particles will be cleared to the oropharynx by the mucociliary apparatus. Soluble particles will be either absorbed into the blood stream directly or pass through the lymphatic system. Insoluble particles, until cleared from the respiratory tract, will continue to irradiate surrounding tissues. In the alveoli, fibrosis and scarring are more likely to occur due to the localized inflammatory response.

All swallowed radioactive material will be handled like any other element in the digestive tract. Absorption depends on the chemical makeup of the contaminant and its solubility. For example, radioiodine and cesium are rapidly absorbed; plutonium, radium, and strontium are not. The lower GI tract is considered the target organ for ingested insoluble radionuclides that pass unchanged in the feces.

The skin is impermeable to most radionuclides. Wounds and burns create a portal for any particulate contamination to bypass the epithelial barrier. All wounds must therefore be meticulously cleaned and debrided when they occur in a radiological environment. Any fluid in the wound may hide weak beta and alpha emissions from detectors.

Once a radionuclide is absorbed, it crosses capillary membranes through passive and active diffusion mechanisms and then is distributed throughout the body. The rate of distribution to each organ is related to organ metabolism, the ease of chemical transport, and the affinity of the radionuclide for chemicals within the organ. The liver, kidney, adipose tissue, and bone have higher capacities for binding radionuclides due to their high protein and lipid makeup.

Protection From Hazards

Forces operating in a theater with nuclear power reactors may be at risk if enemy forces target these reactors and containment facilities. Downwind service members could internalize significant amounts of iodine-131 and other fission byproducts.

MOPP equipment will provide more than adequate protection from radiological contamination. The standard NBC (nuclear, biological, chemical) protective mask will prevent inhalation of any particulate contamination. After prolonged use in a contaminated area, filters should be checked with a radiac prior to disposal.

Normal hospital barrier clothing will provide satisfactory emergency protection for hospital personnel. Ideally, personnel attending a contaminated patient prior to his decontamination will wear anticontamination coveralls. After decontamination, no special clothing is indicated for medical personnel, as the patient presents no risk to medical care providers. In a deployed environment, chemical protective overgarments can be substituted for commercial anticontamination coveralls.

Medical Management

Treatment of internal contamination reduces the absorbed radiation dose and the risk of future biological effects. Administration of diluting and blocking agents enhances elimination rates of radionuclides. Treatment with mobilizing or chelating agents should be initiated as soon as practical when the probable exposure is judged to be significant. Gastric lavage and emetics can be used to empty the stomach promptly and completely after the ingestion of poisonous materials. Purgatives, laxatives, and enemas can reduce the residence time of radioactive materials in the colon.

Ion exchange resins limit gastrointestinal uptake of ingested or inhaled radionuclides. Ferric ferrocyanide (Prussian blue; an investigational new drug, IND) and alginates have been used in humans to accelerate fecal excretion of cesium-137.

Blocking agents, such as stable iodide compounds, must be given as soon as possible after the exposure to radioiodine. A dose of 300 mg of iodide, as administered by a dose of 390 mg potassium iodide, blocks the uptake of radioiodine. When administered prior to exposure to radioiodine, 130 mg of daily oral potassium iodide will suffice. See table 5.

Table 5. Recommended prophylactic single doses of stable iodine.

Age group	Mass of total iodine	Mass of KI	Mass of KIO^3	Volume of Lugol's solution
Adults/adolescents (over 12 yr)	100 mg	130 mg	170 mg	0.8 ml
Children (3–12 yr)	50 mg	65 mg	85 mg	0.4 ml
Infants (1 mo to 3 yr)	25 mg	32.5 mg	42.5 mg	0.2 ml
Neonates (birth to 1 mo)	12.5 mg	16 mg	21 mg	0.1 ml

Mobilizing agents are more effective the sooner they are given after the exposure to the isotope. Propylthiouracil or methimazole may reduce the thyroid's retention of radioiodine. Increasing oral fluids increases tritium excretion.

Chelation agents may be used to remove many metals from the body. Calcium edetate (EDTA) is used primarily to treat lead poisoning but must be used with extreme caution in patients with preexisting renal disease. Diethylenetriaminepentaacetic acid (DTPA, an IND) is more effective in removing many of the heavy-metal, multivalent radionuclides.

The chelates are water soluble and excreted in urine. DTPA metal complexes are more stable than those of EDTA and are less likely to release the radionuclide before excretion. Repeated use of the calcium salt can deplete zinc and cause trace metal deficiencies. Dimercaprol forms stable chelates with mercury, lead, arsenic, gold, bismuth, chromium, and nickel and therefore may be considered for the treatment of internal contamination with the radioisotopes of these elements. Penicillamine chelates copper, iron, mercury, lead, gold, and possibly other heavy metals.

DEPLETED URANIUM

Depleted uranium (DU) is neither a radiological nor chemical threat. It is not a weapon of mass destruction. It is contained in this manual for medical treatment issues. DU is defined as uranium metal in which the concentration of uranium-235 has been reduced from the 0.7% that occurs naturally to a value less than 0.2%. DU is a heavy, silvery-white metal, a little softer than steel, ductile, and slightly paramagnetic. In air, DU develops a layer of oxide that gives it a dull black color.

DU is useful in kinetic-energy penetrator munitions as it is also pyrophoric and literally ignites and sharpens under the extreme pressures and temperatures generated by impact. (The fact that tungsten penetrators do not sharpen on impact—but in fact mushroom—is one reason they are less effective for overcoming armor.) As the penetrator enters the crew compartment of the target vehicle, it brings with it a spray of molten metal as well as shards of both penetrator and vehicle armor (spall), any of which can cause secondary explosions in stored ammunition.

After such a penetration, the interior of the struck vehicle will be contaminated with DU dust and fragments and with other materials generated from armor and burning interior components. Consequently, casualties may exhibit burns derived from the initial penetration as well as from secondary fires. They also may have been wounded by and retain fragments of DU and other metals. Inhalation injury may occur from any of the compounds generated from metals, plastics, and components fused during the fire and explosion.

Wounds that contain DU may develop cystic lesions that solubilize and allow the absorption of the uranium metal. This was demonstrated in veterans of the Persian Gulf War who were wounded by DU fragments. Studies in scientific models have demonstrated that uranium will slowly be distributed systemically with primary deposition in the bone and kidneys from these wounds.

Radiation from DU

DU emits alpha, beta, and weak gamma radiation. Due to the metal's high density, much of the radiation never reaches the surface of the metal. It is thus "self-shielding." Uranium-238, thorium-234, and protactinium-234 will be the most abundant isotopes present in a DU-ammunition round and its fragments.

Intact DU rounds and armor are packaged to provide sufficient shielding to stop the beta and alpha radiations. Gamma-radiation exposure is minimal; crew exposures could exceed limits for the U.S. general population (1 mSv) after several months of continuous operations in an armored vehicle completely loaded with DU munitions. The maximum annual exposure allowed for U.S. radiation workers is 50 mSv. Collection of expended DU munitions and fragments as souvenirs cannot be allowed.

Internalized DU

Internalization of DU through inhalation of particles in dust and smoke, ingestion of particles, or wound contamination present potential radiological and toxicological risks. Single exposures of 1 to 3 μg of uranium per gram of kidney can cause irreparable damage to the kidneys. Skeletal and renal deposition of uranium occurs from implanted DU fragments. The toxic level for long-term chronic exposure to internal uranium metal is unknown, but no renal damage has been documented to date in test models or Gulf War casualties.

The heavy-metal hazards are probably more significant than the radiological hazards. For insoluble compounds, the ingestion hazards are minimal because most of the uranium will be passed through the gastrointestinal tract unchanged. This may not be the case with inhaled DU, as heavy metal may be its primary damaging modality. The normally issued chemical protective mask will provide excellent protection against both inhalation and ingestion of DU particles.

Treatment

Sodium bicarbonate makes the uranyl ion less nephrotoxic. Tubular diuretics may be beneficial. DU fragments in wounds should be removed whenever possible. Laboratory evaluation should include urinalysis, 24-hour urine for uranium bioassay, serum BUN creatinine, beta-

2-microglobulin, creatinine clearance, and liver function studies.

Management of DU Fragments in Wounds

All fragments greater than 1 cm in diameter should be removed if the surgical procedure is practical. Extensive surgery solely to remove DU fragments is NOT indicated. If DU contamination is suspected, the wound should be thoroughly flushed with irrigating solution.

If a DU fragment is excised after wound healing has occurred, care should be taken to not rupture the pseudocyst that may be encapsulating the DU fragment. In experimental studies, this cyst is filled with a soluble-uranium fluid. Capsule tissue is often firmly adhered to the remaining metal fragment.

BIOLOGICAL DOSIMETRY

Physical dosimeters may misrepresent the actual radiation dose and may not be available in a combat or accident irradiation incident. It is important to assess the biological response to an absorbed dose of ionizing radiation in order to predict the medical consequences. The absorbed dose and the fraction of the body exposed should be determined with the highest degree of accuracy available.

General

Differences of 10% in absorbed dose can produce clearly observable variations in biological response. Hematopoietic recovery in heavily irradiated areas of the body will be possible if a sufficient number of stem cells survive in unirradiated or mildly irradiated portions of the hematopoietic system. Knowledge of the heterogeneity of the absorbed dose is particularly important with respect to medical treatment decisions for patients exhibiting radiation-induced bone-marrow syndrome. Cytokine therapy will stimulate proliferation of spared stem cells, but in cases of whole-body stem-cell sterility, bone-marrow transplant may become necessary.

A crude estimate of absorbed dose can be obtained from the clinical presentation and assessment of the response of actively proliferating cell systems to radiation.

Uncertainties in dose estimates arise largely from the high variability between individuals and other factors such as infection.

Generally, the sensitivity of these bioindicators is poor, and given the transient nature of the signs and symptoms in sublethal doses, their clinical usefulness is limited. Biological dosimetry is recommended to support medical treatment decisions.

Reliable biodosimetry is indicated to validate low-dose exposures in occupational radioprotection cases. The analysis of chromosomal aberrations in peripheral blood lymphocytes is widely used to assess radiation dose. Even in partial-body exposures, chromosome damage is an excellent indicator of the absorbed dose.

Many types of chromosomal aberrations may appear in lymphocytes following exposure to radiation. Dicentrics (chromosomes with two centromeres) are biomarkers for ionizing radiation exposure. The incidence of dicentrics in blood lymphocytes for the general population is 1 in 1×10^3 metaphases. Human T-lymphocytes have a long half-life, and a small proportion of them survives for decades. The frequency of dicentrics following exposure remains fairly stable up to a few weeks. After acute partial-body exposure, the irradiated lymphocytes rapidly mix with unirradiated blood, and equilibrium is reached within 24 hours.

Sample Collection

As soon as practical after the irradiation incident, 10 to

15 ml of peripheral blood from the exposed subject is collected in a heparinized blood collection tube. The blood must be immediately transferred under refrigeration to the cytogenetic laboratory. The blood lymphocytes are then isolated and stimulated to grow in culture. Cell proliferation is arrested in the first metaphase, and metaphase spreads are prepared. The stained metaphase spreads are observed under a microscope for enumerating dicentrics.

Observed levels of dicentrics in an exposed individual can then be related to dose by use of an established dose-response calibration curve.

OPERATIONAL ASPECTS

COMMAND RADIATION EXPOSURE GUIDANCE

Line commanders will require advice from their medical officers concerning radiation effects on their personnel. Medical advice must be practical, based upon both the requirements of the mission and the diversity of human response to radiation.

Overreaction to contamination could make the enemy use of an RDD more tenable. The effects of radiation that exceeds normal occupational exposure levels must not be either minimized or exaggerated. NBC risks must be in their proper places relative to the other hazards of combat. Widespread environmental radiological contamination can never be so great as to preclude mandatory mission accomplishment.

Operations Other Than War

Terrorist nuclear weapon use would probably occur without warning. After a ground burst, the area of detonation would be heavily contaminated and would require demarcation until sufficient radionuclide decay occurred.

Areas of contamination from industrial or medical

source destruction, radioactive waste disposal, or use of an RDD could occur. Medical guidance to the commander should be based on long-term effects, primarily increased lifetime cancer risk, of exposure to radiation above normal occupational levels. Current guidelines indicate a 0.008% increase in lifetime risk of fatal cancer per milligray of gamma-radiation exposure. Therefore, an individual who is exposed to 100 mGy (20 times the U.S. occupational annual limit of 0.005 Gy) has an 0.8% increase in lifetime risk of death from cancer.

Allied Command Europe Directive 80–63 defines the measures to be taken against the health hazards of low-level radiation. Such health hazards should not significantly impact the operation per se but rather contribute to the risk of developing long-term health problems.

Operations During War

With exposures below 1.25 Gy, the overall effectiveness of combat units will not be degraded. However, above this threshold, tactical commanders must be advised of their forces' diminished capability to fight.

The term "combat effective" is used for personnel who will be suffering radiation sickness signs and symptoms to a limited degree and who will be able to maintain their performance at at least 75% of their preexposure performance level. Those individuals who are predicted to be "performance degraded" would be operating at a performance level between 25% and 75% of their preexposure performance. Those predicted as "combat ineffective" should be considered as capable of performing their tasks at 25% (at best) of their preexposure performance level.

Adjustment of Unit Radiation Exposure Status

The radiation exposure status (RES) of a given unit is based on the operational exposure above normal background radiation. It is designed to be an average, based upon unit-level dosimeters, and is not useful for the individual casualty.

RES 0	< 0.5 mGy
RES 1A	0.5 to 5 mGy
RES 1B	5 to 50 mGy
RES 1C	50 to 100 mGy
RES 1D	100 to 250 mGy
RES 1E	250 to 750 mGy
RES 2	0.75 to 1.5 Gy
RES 3	> 1.5 Gy

Medical officers may adjust a unit's RES after careful evaluation of the exact exposure status of individual members of the unit. When possible, both physical and biological dosimetry should be used in this regard. The unit status should reflect the arithmetic mode of the available radiation exposure history of all individual members. Any unit member whose exposure status is more than one full category (or subcategory in OOTW) greater than the mode should be replaced. A command health physicist should be consulted whenever possible.

When the exposure dose rate is known to be less than 50 mGy per day, repair of injury is enhanced and the time for cellular repair reduced. Dosimetry should be available in these circumstances that would allow the RES category to be reduced after 3 months at normal background levels.

When individual dosimetry is unavailable, a period of 6 months since the last radiation exposure above background is sufficient to upgrade a unit's RES status one category (or subcategory) one time only. Table 6 shows the effects of exposures from RES 0 through 1E. See appendix C for effects of doses in the nuclear war level.

Table 6. Radiation injuries and effects of radiation exposure of personnel.

RES	Long-term health effects	Medical note	Medical actions
0	Normal risk	U.S. baseline 20% lifetime risk of fatal cancer.	Record in Exposure Record of normally monitored personnel.
1A	Up to 0.04% increased risk of lifetime fatal cancer	None (0.001 Sv annual general pop. exposure limit).	Record as history in Medical Record —tactical operation exposure.

RES	Long-term health effects	Medical note	Medical actions
1B	Occupational risk 0.04–0.4% increased risk of lifetime cancer	Reassurance (0.05 Sv US annual occupational limit).	Record in Medical Record — tactical operation exposure.
1C	0.4–0.8% increased risk of lifetime fatal cancer	Counsel regarding increased long-term risk. No live virus vaccines x 3 months.	Record in Medical Record—tactical operation exposure.
1D	0.8–2% increased risk of lifetime fatal cancer	Potential for increased morbidity of other injuries or incidental disease. < 2% increased lifetime risk of fatal cancer.	Record in Medical Record—tactical operation exposure. Consider routine evacuation from theater IAW commander's operational guidance.
1E	2–6% increased risk of lifetime fatal cancer	Increased morbidity of other injuries or incidental disease. < 6% increased lifetime risk of fatal cancer.	Record in Medical Record—tactical operational exposure. Consider expedited evacuation from theater IAW commander's operational guidance.

GENERAL ASPECTS OF DECONTAMINATION

Contamination is the deposition of radioactive material to levels above the area's normal background radiation. Decontamination is the removal of radioactive particles to make articles suitable for use.

- Personal decontamination is decontamination of self.
- Casualty decontamination refers to the decontamination of casualties.
- Personnel decontamination usually refers to decontamination of noncasualties.
- Mechanical decontamination involves measures to remove radioactive particulates. An example is the filtering of drinking water.

Radiological decontamination is performed in an identical manner to doctrinal chemical decontamination. The main difference is in timing. Chemical decontamination is an emergency. Radiological decontamination is not.

Decontamination of casualties is an enormous task. The process requires dedication of both large numbers of personnel and large amounts of time. Even with appropriate planning and training, the requirement demands a significant contribution of resources.

Removal of outer clothing and rapid washing of exposed skin and hair removes 95% of contamination. The 0.5% hypochlorite solution used for chemicals will also remove radiological contaminants. Care must be taken to not irritate the skin. If the skin becomes erythematous, some radionuclides can be absorbed directly through the skin. Surgical irrigation solutions should be used in liberal amounts in wounds, the abdomen, and the chest. All such solutions should be removed by suction instead of sponging and wiping. Only copious amounts of water, normal saline, or eye solutions are recommended for the eye. Additional care of contaminated wounds is discussed below.

Radiological particulate transfer is a potential problem that can be resolved by a second deliberate decontamination. Decontamination at the medical treatment facility prevents spread of contamination to areas of the body previously uncontaminated, contamination of personnel assisting the patient, and contamination of the medical facility.

Certification of Decontamination

Careful examination of the body with certified radiacs such as the AN/VDR–2 and the AN/PDR–77 will confirm adequate decontamination. Particular attention must be paid to the hands, fingers, face, hair, and feet. For alpha emitters, a count of < 1000 disintegrations/minute and for beta radiation < 1 mR/hour (10 μSv/hour) is clean. Gamma radiation may be detectable at up to twice the local background levels in the decontaminated individual.

Decontamination of Patients

Routine patient decontamination is performed under the supervision of medical personnel. Moist cotton swabs of the nasal mucosa from both sides of the nose should be obtained, labeled, and sealed in separate bags. These swabs can be examined for evidence of radioactive particle inhalation. Significant decontamination will occur in the normal emergency evaluation of patients by careful removal and bagging of clothing.

If practical, skin washwater should be contained and held for disposal. If this water cannot be collected, flushing down standard drains is appropriate. Local water purification units should be notified of this action.

Contaminated tourniquets are replaced with clean ones, and the sites of the original tourniquets are decontaminated. Splints are thoroughly decontaminated, but removed only by a physician. The new dressings are removed in the operating room, placed in a plastic bag, and sealed. Wounds should be covered when adjacent skin is decontaminated so skin contaminants do not enter the wound.

Wound Decontamination

All casualties entering a medical unit after experiencing a radiological attack are to be considered contaminated unless there is certification of noncontamination.

The initial management of a casualty contaminated by radiological agents is to perform all immediate life/limb-saving actions without regard to contamination. Removal of MOPP and other exterior garments during the course of resuscitation will remove nearly all contamination except where the suit has been breached.

Initial Decontamination

During initial decontamination in the receiving areas, bandages are removed and the wounds are flushed; the bandages are replaced only if bleeding recurs.

General Considerations

Only highly energetic gamma emitters present any immediate hazard in wound contamination. It is impossible for a living patient to be so contaminated as to pose a threat to medical providers. Local wound contamination is by particulate matter that should be removed if possible. Alpha and beta emitters left in the wound will cause extensive local damage and may be absorbed into the systemic circulation and redistributed as internal contaminants. If possible, the glove-covered radiac probe should be carefully placed into the dried wound, without touching any of the wound surfaces. DO NOT CONTAMINATE THE PROBE with radioactive particles, body fluids, or talcum powder! Tissue fluids or protective gloves may prevent the detection of alpha and weak beta particles.

After determination that adequate decontamination has been obtained, the wound should again be thoroughly irrigated with saline or other physiologic solution.

Aggressive surgery such as amputation or extensive exploration should not be undertaken to "eliminate radioactive contamination." The surgical damage will far exceed any potential decrease in lifetime radiological exposure risk.

Partial-thickness burns should be thoroughly irrigated and cleaned with mild solutions to minimize irritation of the burned skin. Blisters should be left closed; open blisters should be irrigated and treated in accordance with appropriate burn protocols. In full-thickness burns, radioactive contaminants will slough in the eschar. As there is no circulation in the burned tissue, contaminants will remain in the layers of dead tissue.

Excision of wounds is appropriate when surgically reasonable. Radioactive contaminants will be in the wound surfaces and will be removed with the tissue.

Decontamination of Equipment

In most cases of contamination of equipment and buildings, a mixture of normal housecleaning methods will remove the material. Vacuum cleaners that can handle wet material and have high-efficiency filters are particularly useful. Some surfaces may require repeated scrubbing and vacuuming before they are free of contamination.

Management of Contamination

Personnel Precautions

Protective Masks

Standard issue chemical protective masks afford excellent protection from inhalation and ingestion of radioactive material. Radon and tritium gas will pass through the filters, but short exposures are not medically significant. Increasing oral fluids and maintaining sufficient urine output will adequately treat tritium exposures. Vehicle fires produce dangerous chemical fumes from burning metals and plastics and deplete closed-space oxygen; self-contained breathing apparatus may be necessary in such cases.

Protective Clothing

Commercial anticontamination suits (Tyvek® Anti-C Suits) are ideal but offer little advantage over standard MOPP–4. Chemical-protective overgarments provide excellent contamination protection as well as protection from chemical-biological agents in the combat environment. Standard hospital barrier clothing as used in Universal Precautions is adequate for emergency treatment of limited numbers of radiologically contaminated casualties. Medical personnel should be decontaminated following patients' emergency treatment and decontamination.

Radiac Instruments

The AN/VDR–2 and the AN/PDR–77 are state-of-the-art standard issue radiacs available for issue from the U.S. Army Communications-Electronics Command, Fort Monmouth, NJ 07703–5016.

- **AN/VDR–2: NSN 6665–01–222–1425 $948** Measures gamma dose rates from 0.01 µGy/hour to 99 Gy/hour and beta dose rates from 0.01 milli-roentgen (mR)/hour to 4 R/hour. Functions simultaneously as a dose-rate meter and dose meter, with independent adjustable alarms that can be set at any level over the entire range of each function. Measures total integrated dose to 10 Gy. Dose data are independently stored in a memory for display on command and may be retained when the unit is turned off. Power: Three 9-volt batteries, BA 3090. Size: Instrument, 4 in x 1¾ in x 6⅜ in; Probe, 1½ in x 1½ in x 6¼ in. By Nuclear Research Corporation, Warrington, PA.

- **AN/PDR–77: NSN 6665–01–347–6100 $4500** A portable alpha monitoring and survey device equipped with a 100-cm^2 alpha scintillation probe. Measures alpha radiation from 0 to 999 kilocounts/minute. Includes a digital radiacmeter equipped with full auto-ranging, a user settable dose alarm, built-in test software, a gamma probe identical to the DT–616/VDR–2, and a 5-in diameter x-ray probe. The radiacmeter (with the alpha probe attached) is calibrated using the AN/UDM–6. The radiacmeter and the three interchangeable probes are all contained in a small transit case. Power: Three 9-volt batteries. Replaces both the AN/PDR–56F and the AN/PDR–60. By Nuclear Research Corporation of Warrington, PA.

- **ADM–300A: NSN 6665–01–320–4712 $5249** Detects and quantifies alpha, beta, gamma, and x-ray radiation by using interchangeable probes. Also contains two internal GM tubes. Measures dose rates from 10 μR/hour to 10,000 R/hour gamma and 10 μR/hour to 5 R/hour beta. Accumulated dose can be measured from 1 μR to 1,000 R. Size: 4.5 in x 8.5 in x 2 in; weight: 3 lb.

The 100 cm^2 alpha scintillation probe (AP–100) has an efficiency of 36% and a range of 0 CPM to 1,200,000 CPM. Size: 5 in x 12 in x 3.5 in; weight: 2 lb.

The beta probe (BP–100) is a "pancake" GM tube detector. Automatic background gamma compensation is provided by the internal low-range GM tube. Measures beta contamination to levels of 4 Bq/cm^2 in the presence of high background gamma. Size: 3 in x 11 in x 2.5 in; weight: 12 oz.

The x-ray probe is calibrated to L-shell x-ray emissions from transuranic elements (17 keV) and is designed to detect gross contamination under cover of dust, snow, etc., where alpha detectors would not be practical. Size: 3-in diameter x 6 in; weight: 5.5 oz.

Optional Equipment

- Ion Chamber Probe (under development): Provides gamma measurements from 1 μR/hour through 10 R/hour and is designed for energy emissions > 50 keV. Size: 3-in diameter x 6 in; weight: 5.5 oz.
- Neutron Probe: A BF_3 proportional counter with a range from 0 to 20 rem/hour. Moderator/attenuator design provides dose response corresponding to the human body and provides true rem/hour independent of neutron energies from 0.025 MeV to 15 MeV. Size: 10-in diameter x 12 in; weight: 5 lb.

APPENDICES

A: Table for Medical Assay of the Radiological Patient

B: Table of Internal Contaminant Radionuclides

C: Table of Medical Aspects of Radiation Injury in Nuclear War

D: Decontamination Procedures

E: Biological Dosimetry—On-Site Specimen Collection Procedure

F: Radioactive Materials of Military Significance

G: International System of Units—Conversions

Appendix A: Table for Medical Assay of the Radiological Patient

Test/location	Decon point	Medic. treat. unit (role 2)	Hospital (role 3)	Tertiary care (role 4)
Nasal swabs for inhalation of contaminants	+			
External contamination	+	+	+	
Urine and stool sample for internal contamination		Base-line sample	24-h sample	+
CBC*/platelets		Daily	Daily x 1 wk	Daily x 1 wk
Absolute lymphocyte count		Every 12 h	Every 12 h x 3 d	
HLA† subtyping		Draw sample	Draw sample before lymphocyte count falls	Draw sample before lymphocyte count falls
Cytomegalovirus			+	+
Hemoglobin agglutinin			+	+

Test/location	Decon point	Medic. treat. unit (role 2)	Hospital (role 3)	Tertiary care (role 4)
Human syncytial cell virus antibodies				+
Human immunovirus			+	+
Vesiculovirus				+
Lymphocyte cytogenetics		Draw sample and send forward	Draw sample before lymphocyte count falls	+

*CBC = complete blood count
†HLA = human leucocyte antigen

Appendix B: Table of Internal Contaminant Radionuclides

Element	Respiratory absorption, deposition	GI absorption, deposition	Skin wound absorption	Primary toxicity	Treatment
^{241}Am	75% absorbed 10% retained	Minimal, usually insoluble	Rapid in first few days	Skeletal deposition Marrow suppres-sion Hepatic deposition	Chelation with DTPA or EDTA
$^{137-134}Ce$	Completely absorbed Follows potassium	Com-pletely absorbed Follows potassium	Com-pletely absorbed Follows potassium	Renal excretion Beta and gamma emissions	Ion exchange resins Prussian blue
^{60}Co	High absorption Limited retention	< 5% absorption	Unknown	Gamma emitter	Gastric lavage Penicilla-mine in se-vere cases
^{131}I	High absorption Limited retention	High absorption Limited retention	High absorption Limited retention	Thyroid ablation/ carcinoma	Iodine therapy
^{32}P	High absorption Limited retention	High absorption Limited retention	High absorption Limited retention	Bone, rapidly replicating cells	Lavage, Aluminum hydroxide Phosphates
$^{238-239}Pu$ metal or salt	High absorption Limited retention	Minimal, usually insoluble	Limited absorption May form nodules	Lung, bone, liver	Chelation with DTPA or EDTA

Element	Respiratory absorption, deposition	GI absorption, deposition	Skin wound absorption	Primary toxicity	Treatment
$^{238\text{-}239}Pu$ High-fired oxides	Limited absorption High retention	Minimal, usually insoluble	Limited absorption May form nodules	Local effects from retention in lung	Chelation with DTPA or EDTA Pulmonary lavage*
^{210}Po	Moderate absorption Moderate retention	Minimal	Moderate absorption	Spleen, kidney	Lavage Dimer-caprol
^{226}Ra	Unknown	30% absorption, but 95% fecal excretion	Unknown	Skeletal deposition Marrow suppres-sion Sarcoma	$MgSO_4$ lavage Ammo-nium chloride Calcium Alginates
^{90}Sr	Limited retention	Moderate absorption	Unknown	Bone – follows calcium	Strontium Calcium Ammo-nium chloride
Tritium (T or ^3H) Hydro-gen-3 Tritiated water = HTO	HT – minimal HTO – complete	HT – minimal HTO – complete	HTO – complete	Panmyelo-cytopenia	Dilution with controlled water intake, Diuresis

Element	Respiratory absorption, deposition	GI absorption, deposition	Skin wound absorption	Primary toxicity	Treatment
$^{238-235}U$ fluorides UO_3, sulfates, carbonates	High absorption High retention	High absorption	High absorption Skin irritant	Renal, urinary excretion	Chelation with DTPA* or EDTA $NaHCO^3$
$^{238-235}U$ Some oxides, nitrates	Moderate absorption High retention	Moderate absorption	Unknown	Nephro-toxic Urinary excretion	Chelation with DTPA* or EDTA $NaHCO^3$
$^{238-235}U$ High oxides, hydrides, carbides, salvage ash	Minimal absorption Retention based on particle size	Minimal absorption High excretion	Unknown	Nephro-toxic Urinary excretion	Chelation with DTPA* or EDTA $NaHCO^3$
^{228}U Depleted uranium metal	Retention based on particle size	Minimal absorption High excretion	Forms pseudo-cysts with urinary excretion Limited absorption	Nephro-toxic Deposits in bone, kidney, brain	Particulate removal when possible

* Treatment is not approved by the Food and Drug Administration. Clinical investigations have not begun in the United States.

Appendix C: Table of Medical Aspects of Radiation Injury in Nuclear War

Radiation exposure status (RES) categories and corresponding dose estimates are for comparison purposes only. RES is a maneuver-unit dose designator and is not assigned to an individual.

Combat effective (CE) = > 75% of full capacity
Partially degraded (PD) = 25%–75% of full capacity
Combat ineffective (CI) = < 25% of full capacity

Demanding task (DT) = heavy physical work
Undemanding task (UT) = Sedentary or cognitive work

See Command Radiation Exposure Guidance, page 59, for medical aspects of low-dose radiation.

Dose (est.) Perform-ance capability	Initial symptoms	Initial symptoms interval Onset-End	Antiemetic pretreat-ment effect	Medical problems
0–0.35 Gy CE *Unit RES 1*	None	N/A	Dry mouth Headache	Anxiety
0.35–0.75 Gy CE *Unit RES 1*	Nausea Mild headache	ONSET 6 h END 12 h	Not determined	None
0.75–1.25 Gy CE No further radiation exposure allowable *Unit RES 2*	Transient mild nausea Vomiting in 5–30% of personnel	ONSET 3–5 h END 24 h	5–30% of personnel nauseated without emesis	Potential for delayed traumatic and surgical wound healing Minimal clinical effect

Indicated medical treatment	Disposition without medical care	Disposition with medical care	Clinical remarks
Reassurance Counsel at redeploy-ment	Duty	Duty	Potential for combat anxiety manifestation
Reassurance Counsel at redeploy-ment	Duty	Duty	Mild lymphocyte depression within 24 h
Debride-ment and primary closure of any and all wounds No delayed surgery	Restricted duty No further radiation exposure, elective surgery, or wounding	Restricted duty No further radiation exposure	Moderate drop in lymphocyte, platelet, and granulocyte counts Increased susceptibility to opportunistic pathogens

Dose (est.) Performance capability	Initial symptoms	Initial symptoms interval Onset-End	Antiemetic pretreatment effect	Medical problems
1.25–3 Gy DT: PD from 4 h until recovery UT: PD from 6 h until 1 d and from 6 wk until recovery UT: CE from 1 d to 6 wk *Unit RES 3*	Transient mild to moderate nausea and vomiting in 20–70% of personnel Mild to moderate fatigability and weakness in 25–60% of personnel	ONSET 2–3 h END 2 d	Decreased vomiting Early return to duty for UT Possible increase of fatigability	Significant medical care may be required at 3–5 wk for 10–50% of personnel Anticipated problems should include infection, bleeding, and fever. Wounding or burns will geometrically increase morbidity and mortality.

Indicated medical treatment	Disposition without medical care	Disposition with medical care	Clinical remarks
Fluid and electrolytes for GI losses Consider cytokines for immunocompromised patients (follow granulocyte counts)	LD_5 to LD_{10} Restricted duty No further radiation exposure, elective surgery, or wounding May require delayed evacuation from theater during nuclear war IAW command guidance	Restricted duty No further radiation exposure, elective surgery, or wounding	If there are more than 1.7×10^9 lymphocytes per liter 48 h after exposure, it is unlikely that an individual received a fatal dose. Patients with low (300–500) or decreasing lymphocyte counts or low granulocyte counts should be considered for cytokine therapy and biologic dosimetry using metaphase analysis where available.

Dose (est.) Perform- ance capability	Initial symptoms	Initial symptoms interval Onset-End	Antiemetic pretreat- ment effect	Medical problems
3–5.3 Gy DT: PD from 3 h until recovery UT: PD from 4 h until 2 d, and 7 d until recovery, then CE from 3–7 d *Unit RES 3*	Transient moderate nausea and vomiting in 50–90% of personnel Early: Mild to moderate fatigability and weakness in 80–100% of personnel	Nausea/ vomiting ONSET 2 h END 3–4 d Diarrhea ONSET 10 d END 2–3 wk	Undeter- mined	Frequent diarrheal stools, anorexia, increased fluid loss, ulceration, death of crypt cells and Peyer's Patch lymphoid tissue Increased infection suscepti- bility during immuno- compro- mised timeframe Bleeding diathesis at 3–4 wk due to mega- karyocyte loss

Indicated medical treatment	Disposition without medical care	Disposition with medical care	Clinical remarks
Fluid and electrolytes for GI losses Consider cytokines for immuno-compro-mised patients (follow granulocyte counts) Specific antibiotic therapy for infections May require GI decon-tamination with quinolones Use alimentary nutrition	LD_{10} to LD_{50} Survivors may be able to return to light duty after 5 wk No further radiation exposure May require delayed evacuation from theater	Increased percentage of survivors may be able to return to duty after 5 wk No further radiation exposure May require evacuation from theater for adequate therapy	Moderate to severe loss of lymphocytes. Follow counts q6h in first few days if possible for prognosis. Moderate loss of granulocytes and platelets. Hair loss after 14 d. Thrombocytopenic purpura appears after 3 wk. Consider cytokine therapy and biologic dosimetry using metaphase analysis where available. Loss of crypt cells and GI barriers may allow pathogenic and opportunistic bacterial infection. Use alimentary nutrition to encourage crypt cell growth. Avoid parenteral nutrition and central intravenous lines. Anticipate anaerobic colonization. All surgical procedures must be accomplished in initial 36–48 h after irradiation. Any additional surgery must be delayed until 6 wk postexposure.

Dose (est.) Performance capability	Initial symptoms	Initial symptoms interval Onset-End	Antiemetic pretreatment effect	Medical problems
5.3–8 Gy DT: PD from 3 h to 3 wk, then CI until death or recovery UT: PD from 4 h to 3 d and 7 d to 4 wk CE from 4–7 d, then CI from 4 wk until death or recovery *Unit RES 3*	Moderate to severe nausea and vomiting in 50–90% of personnel Early: Moderate fatigability and weakness in 80–100% of personnel Frequent diarrhea	ONSET under 1 h END indeterminate May proceed directly to GI syndrome without a break	None	At 10 d to 5 wk, 50–100% of personnel will develop pathogenic and opportunistic infections, bleeding, fever, loss of appetite, GI ulcerations, bloody diarrhea, nausea, severe fluid and electrolyte shifts, third space losses, capillary leak, hypotension

in Nuclear War (continued)

Indicated medical treatment	Disposition without medical care	Disposition with medical care	Clinical remarks
Tertiary level intensive care required to improve survival. Fluid and electrolytes for GI losses. May require transfusion and/or colloids. Cytokines for immunocompromised patients. Specific antibiotic therapy for infections, to include antifungals. Will require GI decontamination with quinolones. Use alimentary nutrition.	LD_{50} to LD_{90} At low end of exposure range, death may occur at 6 wk in more than 50% At high end of exposure range, death may occur in 3–5 wk in 90%	Early evacuation to tertiary level medical center before onset of illness Patients will require extensive reverse isolation to prevent cross contamination and nosocomial infection.	Practically no lymphocytes after 48 h. Severe drop in granulocytes and platelets later. In pure radiation exposure scenarios, these patients will require highest priority evacuation. The latent period between prodromal symptoms and manifest illness may be very short. When this radiation injury is combined with any significant physical trauma, survival rates will approach zero. All surgical procedures must be accomplished in initial 36–48 h after irradiation. Any additional surgery must be delayed until 6 wk postexposure. Partial marrow shielding may complicate bone marrow transplant. Steroid therapy is ineffective.

Dose (est.) Perform-ance capability	Initial symptoms	Initial symptoms interval Onset-End	Antiemetic pretreat-ment effect	Medical problems
8–30+ Gy DT: PD from onset of symptoms, then CI from 3 h until death UT: PD from onset of symptoms, then CI from 7 h until death *Unit RES 3*	Severe nausea, vomiting, fatigability, weakness, dizziness, and dis-orientation Moderate to severe fluid and electrolyte imbalance, hypotension, possible high fever, and sudden vascular collapse	ONSET less than 3 min END death	None	Probable death at 2–3 wk Minimal if any break between prodromal syndrome and manifest illness At high radiation levels, CNS symptoms predomin-ate, with death secondary to cerebral vascular incom-petence.

Indicated medical treatment	Disposition without medical care	Disposition with medical care	Clinical remarks
Supportive therapy in higher dosage ranges Aggressive therapy if pure radiation injury and some evidence of response	LD_{90} to LD_{100} Expectant category	If assets are available, then early evacuation to tertiary level medical center during manifest illness. Patients will require extensive reverse isolation to prevent cross contamination and nosocomial infection. Most patients will remain expectant.	Bone marrow totally depleted within days. Bone-marrow transplant may or may not improve ultimate outcome due to late radiation pneumonitis and fibrotic complications. Even minor wounds may prove ultimately fatal. Aggressive therapy is indicated when resources are available and transport to a tertiary care medical center is possible.

Appendix D: Decontamination Procedures

The primary difference between the mechanics of radiological decontamination and chemical decontamination is the method of monitoring. Setup and containment of waste are performed in the same manner. A living patient cannot be so radiologically contaminated as to present an acute hazard to medical personnel. Life- and limb-saving medical attention should never be delayed because of the presence of radioactive material or contamination. Medical personnel must always be alert to the possibility of combined radiological and chemical agent contamination. The chemical agent can present a significant off-gassing or liquid contamination threat to medical personnel.

Patient Decontamination

Patient decontamination is personnel, time, and equipment intensive. Nevertheless, with a little ingenuity and attention to just a few basic principles, an effective litter (field stretcher) decontamination procedure can be accomplished with minimal cost. The first part of this appendix briefly discusses considerations in establishing a decontamination site, and this is followed by step-by-step procedures.

The decontamination site is part of the medical treatment facility, and the same considerations for establishing the treatment facility apply to the decontamination area. The decontamination area is about 50 yards downwind from the treatment area (i.e., wind blows from the clean treatment area to the dirty decontamination area).

Key Principles

- Wind direction
- Security of the decontamination site
- Area control of the decontamination site
- Litter patient decontamination
- Ambulatory patient decontamination

The important considerations of personnel and equipment requirements are discussed in other publications.

Wind Direction

Wind direction is important because resuspension may be present downwind from a contaminated area (i.e., patient arrival/triage area). Patient decontamination is always performed upwind, or at least not downwind, from the patient arrival area.

The decon site will initially be set up to take advantage of the prevailing wind; however, setup should be adaptable to allow for quick rearrangement when the wind comes from another direction.

If the wind changes direction by more than 45 degrees,

the decontamination site will need to be adjusted accordingly. A wait of 15 to 20 minutes to determine if the change is permanent should precede the move. When the site is moved, it must be moved at least 75 meters upwind from any contaminated area. Personnel working in the old "clean" area when the wind shifts must ensure that all casualties remain masked. This scenario points out that the ideal decon setup should include two separate decon sites approximately 75 meters apart, when possible.

Security of Decon Site

When choosing a decontamination site, the same security considerations must be given as any other site chosen for medical operations. The decontamination site is at the same potential risk from attack as is the actual medical treatment facility.

Area Control of Decon Site

An entry control point (ECP) can be established to control movement of clean and contaminated vehicles to the medical treatment facility (MTF) or the decon site. The ECP should be located at a distance far enough from the MTF to keep resuspension hazard from contaminated vehicles to the minimum.

Traffic control at the decon site involves routing a clearly marked one-way course from the ECP to the decon site. Concertina wire works well to keep personnel in the desired areas, and a clearly marked one-way route helps to ensure that correct entry and exit points are used.

Control of personnel movement is necessary to ensure that contaminated walking personnel do not accidentally contaminate clean areas. The hot line must be secured.

Any person or any equipment leaving the contaminated areas must undergo radiological monitoring to ensure that radioactive contaminants do not enter the clean area.

Litter Patient Decontamination

Personnel

Two people are required per litter patient. These two augmentees will link up with one litter patient in the triage area and work with that same litter patient until handoff at the hot line. These two people conduct both clothing removal and any required skin decontamination. To assist these two augmentees, two other augmentees will be needed: one to assist the first two in picking up the patient from the clothing removal litter and the second to remove the contaminated clothing and litter and to replace it with a clean litter. These four augmentees will conduct all patient decontamination and movement of the patient while wearing MOPP–4 or commercial anticontamination (Tyvek® Anti-C) garments with respiratory protection. Each augmentee should wear a personal dosimeter outside of the protective garments between the waist and the neck. If no contaminants other than radiological are present, then commercial Anti-C suits are better tolerated than MOPP–4.

Personnel working in the patient decon area will be at MOPP–4 (or Anti-C). At least two people from this area will move to the triage area and carry the patient from this area to the first decontamination station.

Procedure

Soap and water are satisfactory decon solutions for radiological hazards. In situations where combined NBC-agent threats are present, chemical decontamination solutions should be used and MOPP–4 maintained.

1. Carefully monitor the patient to determine presence of radiological contamination.
   a. Mark contaminated areas on body diagram.
   b. Scan by moving the radiac slowly over the entire body while maintaining a distance not greater than 10 cm. Do not touch the patient with the radiac.

2. Decontaminate and remove the Quick Doff Hood.
   a. Sponge down front, sides, and top of hood with soap and water or 5% calcium hypochlorite solution.
   b. Rinse scissors.
   c. Cut off hood.
      (1) Release or cut hood shoulder straps.
      (2) Cut/untie neck cord.
      (3) Cut/remove zipper cord.
      (4) Cut/remove drawstring under the voicemitter.
      (5) Unzip the hood zipper.
      (6) Cut the cord away from the mask.

(7) Cut the zipper below voicemitter.
(8) Proceed cutting upward, close to the inlet valve covers and eye lens outserts.
(9) Cut upward to top of eye lens outsert.
(10) Cut across forehead to the outer edge of the next eye lens outsert.
(11) Cut downward toward the patient's shoulder, staying close to the eye lens outsert inlet-valve cover.
(12) Cut across the lower part of the voicemitter to the zipper.
(13) Rinse scissors.
(14) Cut from center of forehead over the top of the head.
(15) Fold left and right sides of the hood to each side of the patient's head, laying sides on the litter.

3. Decontaminate protective mask/face.
   a. Use soap and water or 0.5% hypochlorite.
   b. Cover both inlet valve covers with gauze or hands.
   c. Wipe external parts of mask.
   d. Uncover inlet valve covers.
   e. Wipe exposed areas of the patient's face.
      (1) Chin
      (2) Neck
      (3) Back of ears

4. Remove Field Medical Card (FMC) and personal dosimeter

a. Cut FMC tie wire.
b. Allow FMC to fall into a plastic bag.
c. Seal plastic bag and wash with 0.5% hypochlorite.
d. Place plastic bag under back of mask head straps.
e. Wipe dosimeter with damp cloth and place in separate plastic bag.
f. Replace dosimeter on patient after decon is completed.

5. Remove all gross contamination from patient's overgarment and place it in designated containers. These containers must be removed to a safe location at frequent intervals to decrease the overall dose-rate in the decon area.
   a. Wipe all evident contamination spots with soap and water or 5% hypochlorite.
   b. Wipe mask with soap and water.

6. Cut and remove overgarments. Cut clothing around tourniquets, bandages, and splints. Two persons will be cutting clothing at the same time. Rinse scissors before doing each complete cut to avoid contaminating inner clothing.
   a. Cut overgarment jacket.
      (1) Unzip protective overgarment.
      (2) Cut from wrist area of sleeves, up to armpits, and then to neck area.
      (3) Roll chest sections to respective sides with inner surface outward.
      (4) Tuck clothing between arm and chest.

(5) Repeat procedure for other side of jacket.

b. Cut overgarment trousers.

(1) Cut from cuff along inseam to waist on left leg.

(2) On right overgarment leg, cut from cuff to just below zipper and then go sideways into the first cut.

(3) Allow trouser halves to drop to litter with contamination away from patient.

(4) Tuck trouser halves to sides of body and roll the camouflage sides under, between the legs.

7. Remove outer gloves. This procedure can be done by two augmentees, one on each side of the patient, working simultaneously. Do not remove inner gloves.

a. Lift the patient's arms by grasping his gloves.

b. Fold the glove away from the patient over the sides of the litter.

c. Grasp the fingers of the glove.

d. Roll the cuff over the finger, turning the glove inside out.

e. Carefully lower the arm(s) across the chest when the glove(s) is removed. Do not allow the arms to contact the exterior (camouflage side) of the overgarment.

f. Dispose of contaminated gloves.

(1) Place in plastic bag.

(2) Deposit in contaminated dump.

g. Rinse your own gloves.

8. Remove overboots.
   a. Cut laces.
   b. Fold lacing eyelets flat outward.
   c. Hold heels with one hand.
   d. Pull overboots downward over the heels with other hand.
   e. Pull toward you until removed.
   f. Place overboots in contaminated disposal bag.

9. Remove personal articles from pockets.
   a. Place in plastic bags.
   b. Seal bags.
   c. Place bags in contaminated holding area.

10. Remove combat boots without touching body surfaces.
    a. Cut boot laces along the tongue.
    b. Pull boots downward and toward you until removed.
    c. Place boots in contaminated dump.

11. Remove inner clothing.
    a. Unbuckle belt.
    b. Cut BDU (battle dress uniform) pants following same procedures as for overgarment trousers.
    c. Cut fatigue jacket following same procedures as for overgarment jacket.

12. Remove undergarments following same procedure as for fatigues. If patient is wearing a brassiere, it is cut between cups. Both shoulder straps are cut where they attach to cups and laid back off shoulders.

13. After the clothing has been cut away, transfer the

patient to a decontamination litter or a canvas litter with a plastic sheeting cover.

a. Carefully monitor the patient, paying particular attention to face, hands, feet, and any areas where evidence indicates outer clothing may have been breached.
b. Use a five-member team that, using the buddy system, decontaminates their gloves with soap and water or 5% hypochlorite solution. One member places his hands under the small of the patient's legs and thigh; a second member places his arms under the patient's back and buttocks; and the third member places his arms under the patient's shoulders and supports the head and neck. They carefully lift the patient using their knees, not their backs, to minimize back strain. While the patient is elevated, another decon team member removes the litter from the litter stands and another member replaces it with a decontamination (clean) litter. The patient is carefully lowered onto the clean litter.
c. Two decon members carry the litter to the skin decontamination station.
d. Place the contaminated clothing and overgarments in bags and move them to the decontaminated waste dump.
e. Rinse the dirty litter with the 5% decontamination solution and place it in a litter storage area.
f. Return decontaminated litters by ambulance to the maneuver units.

14. Decontaminate the patient, his wounds, and the stretcher.
    a. Take care to not scrub the skin and cause erythema. The areas of potential contamination should be spot decontaminated using soap and water or 0.5% hypochlorite. These areas include the neck, wrists, lower face, and skin under tears or holes in the protective ensemble.
    b. Change any dressings or tourniquets.
        (1) Flush superficial (not body cavity, eye, or nervous tissue) wounds with the cleansing or irrigation solution and apply new dressings as needed. Cover massive wounds with plastic or plastic bags.
        (2) Place new tourniquets 0.5 to 1 inch proximal to the original tourniquets, then remove the old tourniquets.
        (3) Superficially decontaminate any splint. Do not remove it. If a splint cannot be saturated (air splint or canvas splint), remove it sufficiently so that everything below the splint can be washed.

15. Conduct final contamination monitoring using the radiac, the CAM (chemical agent monitor), M8 paper, or M9 paper. If no chemical contamination is present in the area, only radiological monitoring with the radiac is necessary.

16. Once the patient is confirmed clean of radiological

contaminants and chemical agents, transfer him via a shuffle pit over the hot line and to the treatment area. The shuffle pit is composed of 2 parts supertropical bleach (STB) and 3 parts earth or sand. The shuffle pit should be deep enough to cover the bottom of the protective overboots.

a. If there is a limited supply of decontaminatable stretchers, transfer the patient to a new clean canvas litter. Use the previously described procedures for a five-member team that, using the buddy system, decontaminates their gloves with soap and water or 5% hypochlorite solution and then transfers the patient.
b. Place the patient and litter over the hot line.

Ambulatory Patient Decon

Casualties who are decontaminated in an ambulatory area are those who either require treatment that can be supplied in the emergency treatment area or require resupply of their protective overgarments in the clean area before return to duty. Those who require clothing removal use the litter decontamination procedure, as removal of clothing is not done in this area.

Personnel

Personnel from the decontamination station might assist the casualty, or the casualties might assist each other during this process under close supervision.

Procedure

Decontamination of ambulatory patients follows the same principles as for litter patients. The major difference is the sequence of clothing removal to lessen the chance of patient contaminating himself and others. The first five steps are the same as in litter patient decontamination and are not described in detail.

Initially, monitor the patient with a radiac to confirm the presence of radiological contamination.

1. Remove load-bearing equipment and personal dosimeter.
2. Decontaminate mask and hood and remove hood.
3. Decontaminate skin around mask.
4. Remove Field Medical Card and put it into a plastic bag.
5. Remove gross contamination from the outer garment.
6. Remove and bag personal effects from overgarment.
7. Remove overgarment jacket.
   a. Instruct the patient to
      (1) Clench his fists.
      (2) Stand with arms held straight down.
      (3) Extend arms backward at about a 30-degree angle.
      (4) Place feet shoulder width apart.
   b. Stand in front of the patient.
      (1) Untie drawstring.

(2) Unsnap jacket front flap.
(3) Unzip jacket front.

c. Move to the rear of the patient.
(1) Grasp jacket collar at sides of the neck.
(2) Peel jacket off shoulders at a 30-degree angle down and away from the patient.
(3) Smoothly pull the inside of sleeves over the patient's wrists and hands.

d. Cut to aid removal if necessary.

8. Remove butyl rubber gloves.

a. Patient's arms are still extended backward at a 30-degree angle.
(1) Dip your gloved hands in 5% hypochlorite solution.
(2) Use thumbs and forefingers of both hands.
(a) Grasp the heel of the patient's glove at top and bottom of forearm.
(b) Peel gloves off with a smooth downward motion. This procedure can easily be done with one person or with one person on each side of the patient working simultaneously.
(c) Place gloves in contaminated disposal bag.

b. Tell the patient to reposition his arms but to not touch his trousers.

9. Remove the patient's overboots.

a. Cut overboot laces with scissors dipped in 5% hypochlorite.
b. Fold lacing eyelets flat on ground.
c. Step on the toe and heel eyelet to hold eyelets on the ground.
d. Instruct the patient to step out of the overboot onto clean area. If in good condition, the overboot can be decontaminated and reissued.

10. Remove overgarment trousers.
    a. Unfasten or cut all ties, buttons, or zippers.
    b. Grasp trousers at waist.
    c. Peel trousers down over the patient's boots.
    d. Cut trousers to aid removal if necessary.
        (1) Cut around all bandages and tourniquets.
        (2) Cut from inside pant leg ankle to groin.
        (3) Cut up both sides of the zipper to the waist.
        (4) Allow the narrow strip with zipper to drop between the legs.
        (5) Peel or allow trouser halves to drop to the ground.
    e. Tell the patient to step out of trouser legs one at a time.
    f. Place trousers into contaminated disposal bag.

11. Remove glove inner liners. The patient should remove the liners, since this will reduce the possibility of spreading contamination. Tell the patient to remove white glove liners.
    a. Grasp heel of glove without touching exposed skin.

b. Peel liner downward and off.
c. Drop liner in contaminated disposal.
d. Remove the remaining liner in the same manner.
e. Place liners into contaminated disposal bag.

12. Conduct final monitoring and decontamination.
    a. Monitor/test with radiac.
    b. Check all areas of patient's clothing.
    c. Give particular attention to
        (1) Discolored areas
        (2) Damp spots
        (3) Tears in clothing
        (4) Neck
        (5) Wrist
        (6) Around dressings
    d. Decontaminate all contamination on clothing or skin by cutting away areas of clothing or using soap and water or 5% hypochlorite.
    e. Wipe off personal dosimeter and replace on patient.

13. The medical corpsman should remove bandages and tourniquets and decontaminate splints, using the procedures described in the decontamination of a litter patient, during overgarment removal.

14. After radiac monitoring confirms that the patient is decontaminated, he is ready to move inside the hot line. Instruct the patient to shuffle his feet to dust his boots thoroughly as he walks through the shuffle pit.

In the clean treatment area, the patient can now be re-triaged, treated, evacuated, etc. In a hot climate, the patient will probably be significantly dehydrated, and the rehydration process should start.

Comments

The clean area is the resupply point for the patient decontamination site. Water is needed for rehydration of persons working in the decon area. The resupply section should have an adequate stock of canteens with the chemical cap.

A location is needed in each decon area (75 meters from the working decon site) to allow workers to remove their masks and rehydrate. There are generally not enough BDOs (battle dress overgarments) available to allow workers to remove them during the rest cycle and don new gear before going back to work. If these clean/shaded rest areas are not provided, the workers must remain in MOPP–4 even during rest periods, and water must be drunk through the mask via the drinking port. If all water consumption is by mask, there must be a canteen refill area adjacent to the vapor/clean line in which empty canteens can be deconned and placed for refill and clean full canteens are present for rehydration.

(The above procedures were adapted from Field Manual (FM) 8–10–4, Medical Platoon Leaders' Handbook: Tactics, Techniques, and Procedures; FM 8–10–7, Health Service Support in a Nuclear, Biological, and Chemical

Environment; and the Medical Management of Chemical Casualties Handbook.)

Casualty Receiving Area

The following diagram shows a setup for casualty reception in a contaminated environment. The actual setup of this area may vary depending on the assets and circumstances.

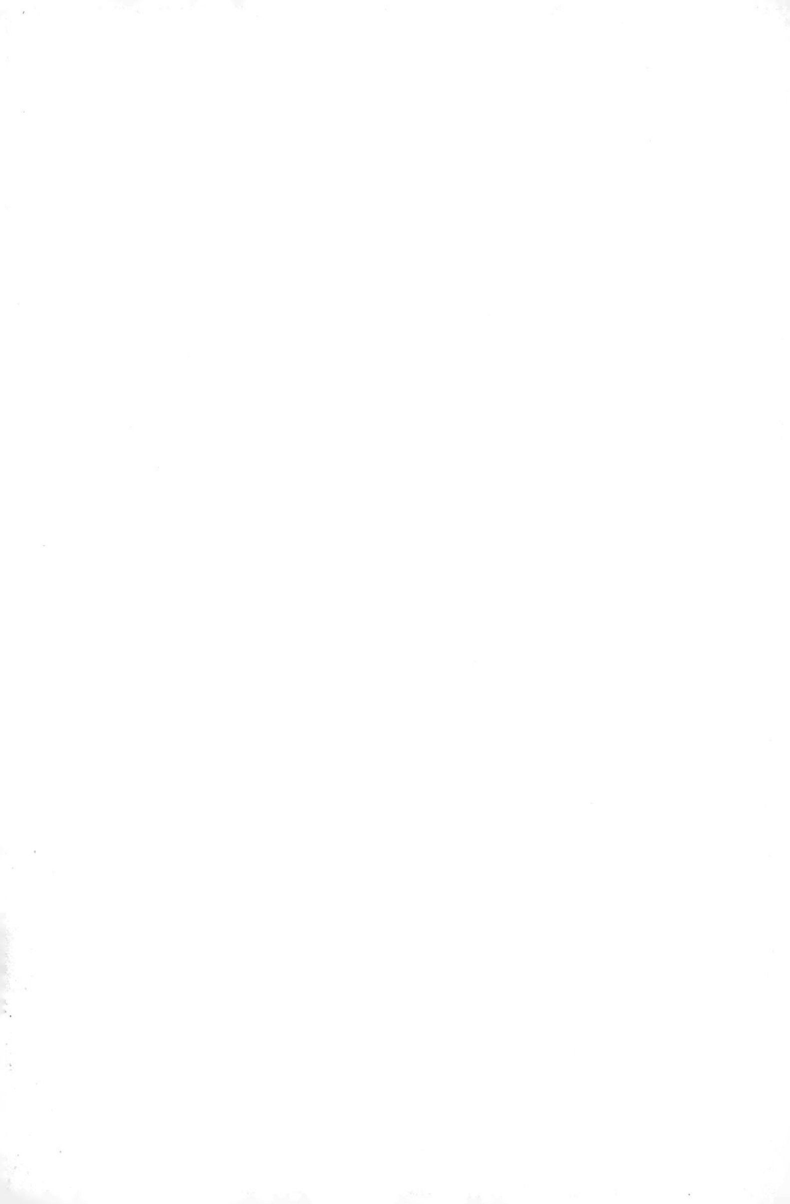

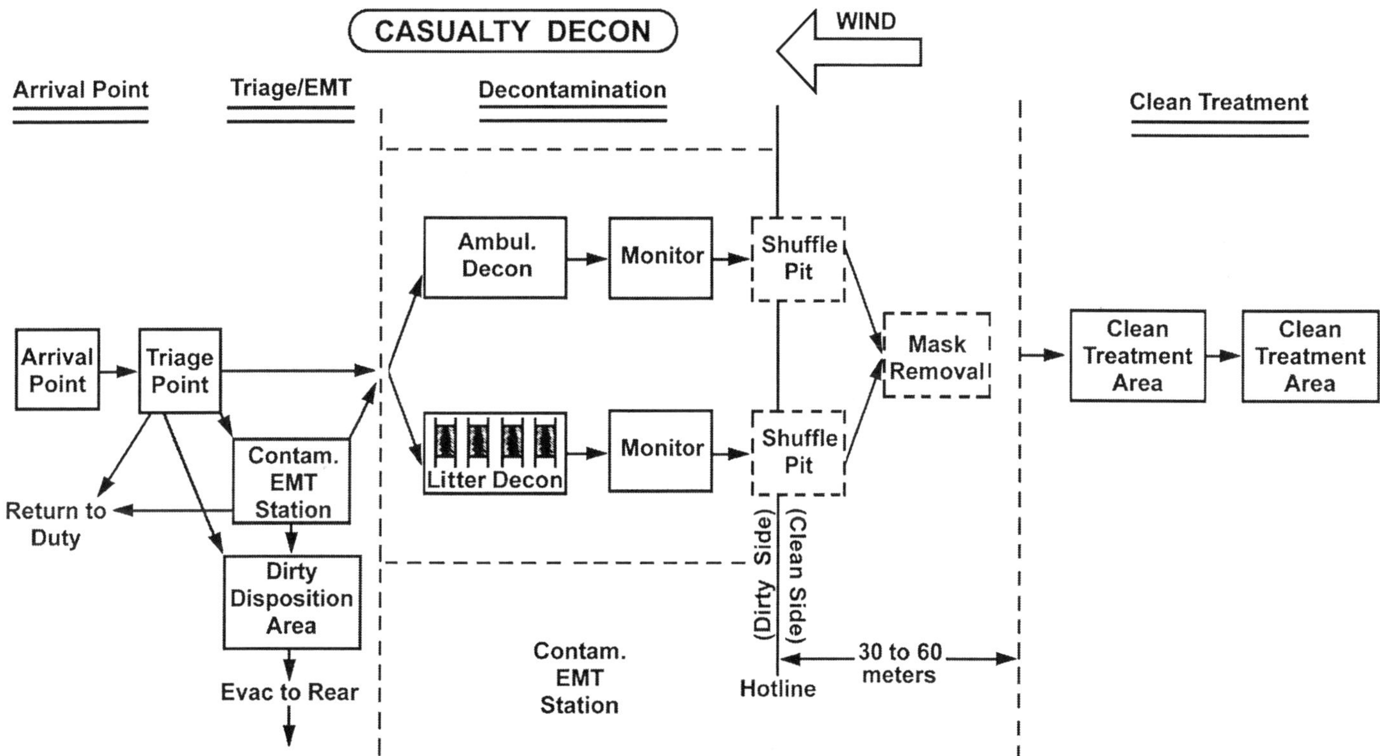
CASUALTY DECON
WIND
Arrival Point
Triage/EMT
Decontamination
Clean Treatment
Arrival Point
Triage Point
Contam. EMT Station
Return to Duty
Dirty Disposition Area
Evac to Rear
Ambul. Decon
Litter Decon
Monitor
Monitor
Shuffle Pit
Shuffle Pit
Mask Removal
Clean Treatment Area
Clean Treatment Area
(Dirty Side)
(Clean Side)
Hotline
30 to 60 meters
Contam. EMT Station

Personnel Decontamination Station

The following foldout is a diagram of a personnel decontamination station. This is a decontamination configuration for *noncasualty* personnel, but its procedures may be used by any military unit.

Contaminated noncasualty personnel use the procedures to move from the contaminated (dirty) area across the hot line to the noncontaminated (clean) area. In a medical unit, the procedures are utilized by personnel working in the dirty area, such as the triage officer and the decontamination team, to move to the clean area.

Related procedures occur in the MOPP exchange station (not shown). In this station, personnel who have been wearing contaminated MOPP gear longer than the recommended time can exchange their dirty protective garments for clean garments.

(This information is from Army Field Manual 3–5 (FM 3–5), Fleet Marine Field Manual No. 11–10 (FMFM 11–10): NBC Decontamination.)

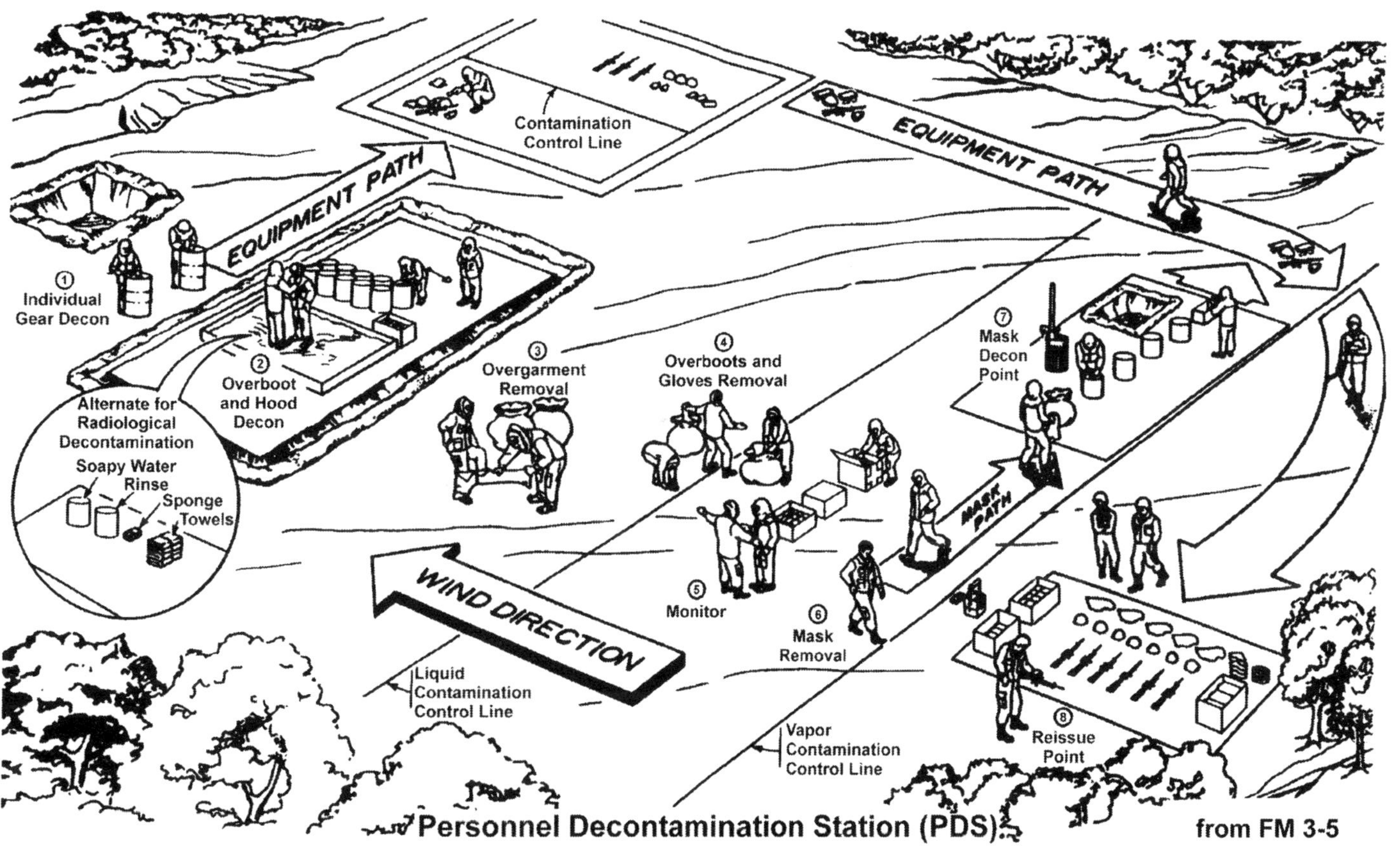

Personnel Decontamination Station (PDS) from FM 3-5

Appendix E: Biological Dosimetry—On-Site Specimen Collection Procedure

Biological dosimetry is a research-based dose assessment tool that can assist the clinician by measuring aberrations in lymphocyte chromatin following exposure to ionizing radiation. It is particularly useful after partial-body exposure in conjunction with physical dosimetry. It can also be useful in validating dose reconstruction when the accidentally exposed individual was not wearing a dosimeter. If at all possible, specimens should be collected before peripheral lymphocyte counts fall and sent to:

Experimental Assays Assessing Radiation Exposure
AFRRI–95–3 Biological and Biophysical
Dosimetry Team
Armed Forces Radiobiology Research Institute
Receiving, Building 42
8901 Wisconsin Avenue
Bethesda, MD 20889–5603, USA

Contact AFRRI Biodosimetry by calling 301–295–0484 or fax 301–295–6567. Alternatively, the Medical Radiobiology Assistance Team (MRAT) physician can be reached at 301–295–0316. AFRRI will discuss the patient and provide by fax an informed consent form. As this is an experimental procedure at this time, only limited numbers of samples can be processed.

To ensure successful accomplishment of cytogenetic tasks, it is important that the cytogenetic laboratory receive blood samples as soon as possible after collection. To expedite freight to AFRRI, coordinate blood sample collection with flight/courier schedules to minimize delay, exposure to extreme temperatures, and exposure to ionizing radiation during transit.

Instructions for Blood Collection

1. Obtain informed consent of the patient and have the consent form filled out and signed; provide a copy to the patient.

2. Coordinate the blood collection time with the shipping/flight schedule to ensure AFRRI's Dosimetry Team will receive the specimen within 32 hours of collection. Use of a courier to transport the package is advisable to assure successful transport.

3. Using a Vacutainer sleeve and sterile needle, draw 4 to 5 tubes of blood (approximately 40 ml) into 8-ml sterile Vacutainers containing heparin, for freight to AFRRI. Label each tube. Several Vacutainers are provided as backups in the event that some tubes lose their vacuum.

4. Immediately after blood collection, gently invert Vacutainer tubes to mix the blood and anticoagulant. Clotted blood samples cannot be used.

5. Blood samples must be KEPT COOL, BUT NOT FROZEN after collection and during shipment.
6. Individually wrap Vacutainers in the protective materials provided and pack in the insulated container. Secure tubes with paper or other coolant packing material to prevent breakage during freight handling.
7. Label the package "DO NOT X-RAY, BIOHAZARD, BIOLOGICAL SAMPLE, FRAGILE."
8. Ship samples as soon as possible for express delivery by courier or special carrier, such as Federal Express or Airborne Express, to AFRRI at the address provided.
9. Notify the AFRRI Biodosimetry Team of the shipping carrier and shipping number ASAP. International shipments should be sent by courier to allow rapid customs transit.

Appendix F: Radioactive Materials of Military Significance

Americium

Cesium

Cobalt

Depleted Uranium

Iodine

Phosphorus

Plutonium

Radium

Strontium

Tritium

Uranium

THE FOLLOWING PAGES MAY BE REMOVED BY TEARING ALONG THE PERFORATIONS.

AMERICIUM

Americium-241 (^{241}Am) is a decay daughter of plutonium and an alpha emitter. It is detectable with a standard radiac such as the FIDLER instrument due to emission of a 60-kEv gamma ray.

It is used in smoke detectors and other instruments, and it will be found in fallout from a nuclear weapon detonation.

It is a heavy metal poison but, in large quantities, can cause whole-body irradiation.

Seventy-five percent of an initial lung burden is absorbed, with 10% of the particles retained in the lung. Gastrointestinal absorption of americium is minimal, but it may be absorbed rapidly from skin wounds.

It is eliminated by urinary and hepatic excretion.

TREATMENT: DTPA or EDTA chelation in the first 24 to 48 hours following pulmonary exposure.

CESIUM

Cesium-137 (^{137}Ce) is commonly found in medical radiotherapy devices. It was used in the Chechen RDD threat against Moscow. The mishandling of a medical radiotherapy device was responsible for the worst radiation accident in the Western Hemisphere. It emits both gamma rays and beta radiation and can be readily detected by gamma instruments. It is completely absorbed by the lungs and GI tract and from wounds. It is soluble in most forms and is treated by metabolism as a potassium analog. Excretion is in urine. Primary toxicity is whole-body irradiation. Deaths due to acute radiation syndrome have occurred.

TREATMENT: Prussian blue (investigational new drug in the United States from Oak Ridge Affiliated Universities, Oak Ridge, TN; available in overseas civilian medical community) and ion exchange resins. If early after ingestion, lavage and purgatives.

COBALT

Cobalt-60 (^{60}Co) is used in medical radiotherapy devices and commercial food irradiators. It will most likely be found after improper disposal, or after destruction of a hospital or commercial facility. It generates high-energy gamma rays and 0.31-MeV beta rays. It is easily detectable with a gamma detector.

Cobalt could be used as a contaminant in an improvised nuclear device to make the fallout more radioactive.

Cobalt will be rapidly absorbed from the lung, but less than 5% will be absorbed from the GI tract. Nothing is known about absorption from wounds. Primary toxicity will be from whole-body irradiation and acute radiation syndrome.

TREATMENT: Gastric lavage, purgatives. Severe cases might be treated by chelation with penicillamine.

DEPLETED URANIUM

Depleted uranium (DU) emits limited alpha, beta, and some gamma radiation. DU does not cause radiation threat. It is found in armor-piercing munitions, armor, and aircraft counterweights. It is readily detectable with a typical end-window G-M (Geiger-Mueller) counter.

Inhaled uranium compounds may be metabolized and result in urinary excretion. Inhalation of DU oxides may occur during tank fires or by entering destroyed armored vehicles without a protective mask. Absorption will be determined by the chemical state of the uranium. Soluble salts are readily absorbed; the metal is not. DU fragments in wounds become encapsulated and are gradually metabolized, resulting in whole-body distribution, particularly to bone and kidney. In laboratory tests, DU does cross the placenta. No renal toxicity has been documented to date.

TREATMENT: Sodium bicarbonate makes the uranyl ion less nephrotoxic. Tubular diuretics may be beneficial. DU fragments in wounds should be removed whenever possible. Extensive surgery solely to remove DU fragments is NOT indicated. All fragments greater than 1 cm in diameter should be removed when the procedure is practical. Laboratory evaluation should include urinalysis, 24-hour urine for uranium bioassay, serum BUN, creatinine, beta-2-microglobulin, creatinine clearance, and liver function studies.

IODINE

Iodine–131, 132, 134, 135 ($^{131, 132, 134, 135}I$) will be found after reactor accidents and following the destruction of a nuclear reactor by hostile forces. Radioactive iodine (RAI) is a normal fission product found in reactor fuel rods. It is released by rupturing the reactor core and its containment vessel. Postdestruction winds will determine the fallout pattern. Most of the radiation is beta rays, with some gamma.

Primary toxicity is to the thyroid gland. Thyroid uptake concentrates the RAI and allows local irradiation similar to therapeutic thyroid ablation. A high incidence of childhood thyroid carcinoma was documented following the Chernobyl disaster.

TREATMENT: If exposure is anticipated, daily administration of 130 mg of sodium or potassium iodide (NaI, KI) will prevent uptake. Postexposure, 300 mg NaI or KI daily x 7 to 10 days will prevent thyroid uptake. Oral propylthiouracil 100 mg q8hours x 8 days or oral methimazole 10 mg q8hours x 2 days, then 5 mg q8hours x 6 days, may also be used.

PHOSPHORUS

Phosphorus-32 (^{32}P) will generally be found in research laboratories and in medical facilities where it is used as a tracer. It has a strong beta ray and can be detected with the beta shield open on a beta-gamma detector.

Phosphorus is completely absorbed from all sites. It is deposited in the bone marrow and other rapidly replicating cells. Local irradiation causes cell damage.

TREATMENT: Lavage, aluminum hydroxide, and oral phosphates.

PLUTONIUM

Plutonium-239, 238 ($^{239, 238}Pu$) is produced from uranium in reactors. It is the primary fissionable material in nuclear weapons and is the predominant radioactive contaminant in nuclear weapons accidents. The primary radiation is in the form of alpha particles, so plutonium does not present an external irradiation hazard. It is always contaminated with americium, which does have a fairly easily detectable x ray by use of a thin-walled gamma probe.

Primary toxicity is from inhalation. Five-micron or smaller particles will remain in the lung and are metabolized based on the salt solubility. Particles that remain will cause local irradiation damage. GI absorption will depend upon the chemical state of the plutonium; the metal is not absorbed. Stool specimens will be positive after 24 hours and urine specimens after 2 weeks. Wound absorption is variable. Plutonium may be washed from intact skin.

TREATMENT: Nebulized or IV: 1 g CaDTPA within 24 hours of exposure; follow by 1 g ZnDTPA qd monitoring urine levels (IND).

RADIUM

Radium-226 (^{226}Ra) is not a federally regulated commodity and has no U.S. military use. It may be encountered in FSU equipment* as instrument illumination, in industrial applications, and in older medical equipment. Primary radiation is alpha particles, but daughter products emit beta and gamma rays and, in quantity, may present a serious external irradiation hazard.

Most exposure is by ingestion, with 30% absorption. Little is known about wound absorption, but radium will follow calcium to bone deposition. Long-term exposure is associated with leukemia, aplastic anemia, and sarcomas.

TREATMENT: Immediate lavage with 10% magnesium sulfate followed by saline and magnesium purgatives after ingestion. Ammonium chloride may increase fecal elimination.

---

* Former Soviet Union (FSU) equipment is manufactured and used by militaries throughout the world as a result of arms purchases and technology transfers.

STRONTIUM

Strontium-90 (^{90}Sr) is a direct fission product (daughter) of uranium. It and its daughters emit both beta and gamma rays and can be an external irradiation hazard if present in quantity.

Strontium will follow calcium and is readily absorbed by both respiratory and GI routes. Up to 50% of a dose will be deposited in bone.

TREATMENT: Immediately after ingestion, oral administration of aluminum phosphate can decrease absorption by as much as 85%. Administration of stable strontium can competitively inhibit the metabolism and increase the excretion of radiostrontium. Large doses of calcium and acidification of the urine with ammonium chloride will also increase excretion.

TRITIUM

Tritium (hydrogen-3 or ^3H) is hydrogen with a nucleus composed of two neutrons and one proton. It is used in nuclear weapons and in U.S. (and other Western) luminescent gun sights and muzzle-velocity detectors. It is unlikely to be a hazard except in a closed space. Tritium gas rapidly diffuses into the atmosphere. Tritium is a beta emitter and is not a significant irradiation hazard.

Water formed from tritium (HTO) is completely absorbed and equilibrates with body water. It is excreted in urine, and urine samples will be positive within an hour of significant exposure. No adverse health effects have been reported from a single exposure.

TREATMENT: The biologic half-time is 10 to 12 days. Increasing oral fluids to tolerance will reduce this by half. Care must be taken to not overhydrate an individual and cause iatrogenic water intoxication.

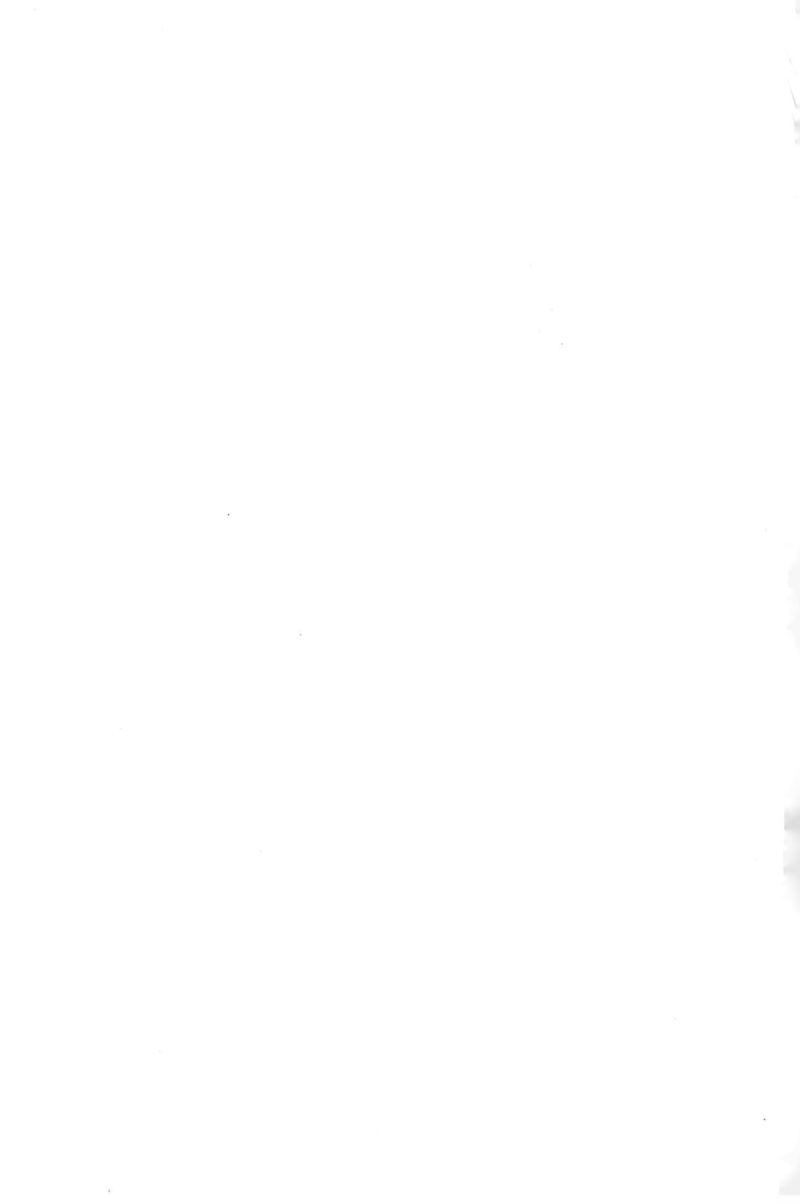

URANIUM

Uranium-238, 235, 239 ($^{238, 235, 239}U$) is found, in order of increasing radioactivity, in depleted uranium (DU), natural uranium, fuel rods, and weapons-grade material. Uranium and its daughters emit alpha, beta, and gamma radiation. DU and natural uranium are not serious irradiation threats. Used fuel rods and weapons-grade (enriched) uranium containing fission products can emit significant levels of gamma. If enough enriched uranium is placed together, a critical mass may form and emit lethal levels of radiation. This could be encountered in a fuel-reprocessing plant or melted reactor core.

Inhaled uranium compounds may be metabolized and excreted in the urine. Urinary levels of 100 μg per deciliter following acute exposure may cause renal failure. Absorption will be determined by the chemical state of the uranium. Soluble salts are readily absorbed; the metal is not.

TREATMENT: Sodium bicarbonate makes the uranyl ion less nephrotoxic. Tubular diuretics may be beneficial. Laboratory evaluation should include urinalysis, 24-hour urine for uranium bioassay, serum BUN creatinine, beta-2-microglobulin, creatinine clearance, and liver function studies.

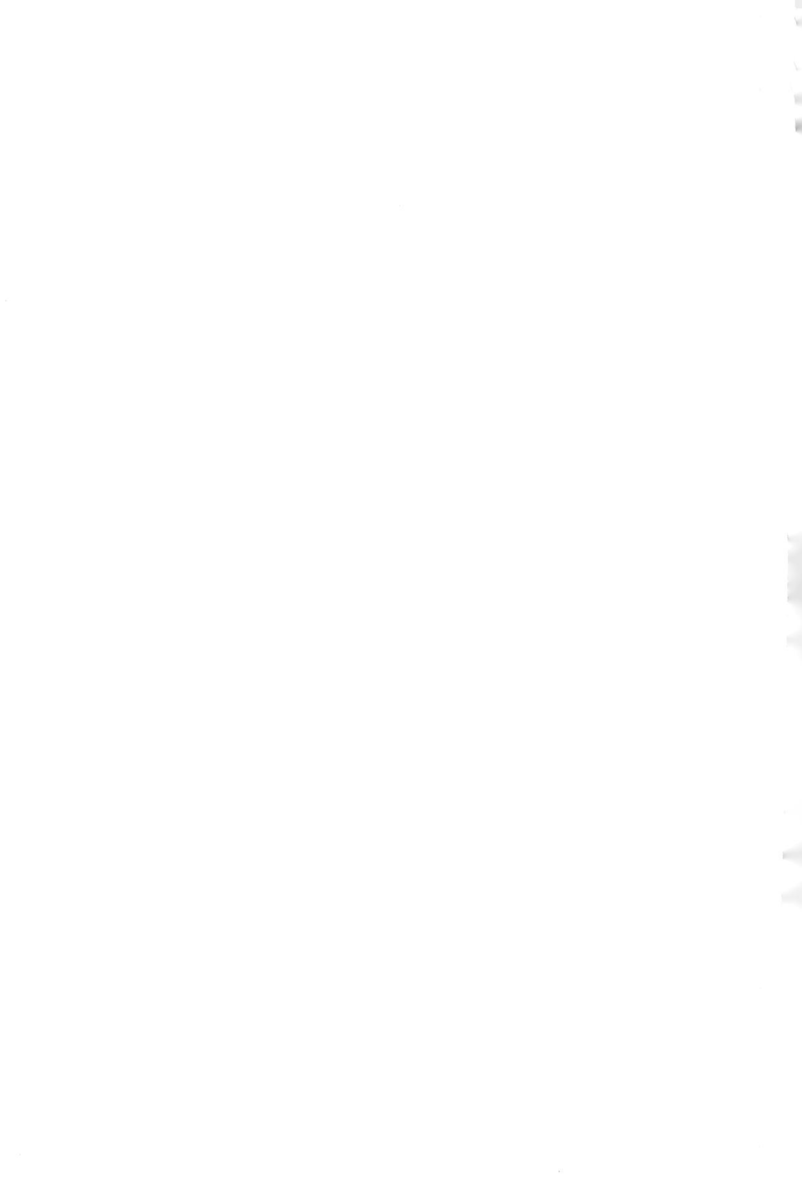

Appendix G. International System of Units—Conversions

Old unit	SI unit	Old unit	SI unit
curie (Ci)	**becquerel (Bq)**	**rem**	**sievert (Sv)**
1 pCi	37 mBq	0.1 mrem	1 μSv
27 pCi	1 Bq	1 mrem	0.01 mSv
1 μCi	37 kBq	1 mrem	10 μSv
27 μCi	1 MBq	100 mrem	1 mSv
1 Ci	37 GBq	500 mrem	5 mSv
27 Ci	1 TBq	1 rem	10 mSv
		1 rem	1 cSv
rad	**gray (Gy)**	100 rem	1 Sv
1 rad	10 mGy		
1 rad	1 cGy		
100 rad	1 Gy		

Symbol	Name	Multiplier	Value
p	pico	10^{-12}	million millionth
n	nano	10^{-9}	thousand millionth
μ	micro	10^{-6}	millionth
m	milli	10^{-3}	thousandth
c	centi	10^{-2}	hundredth
k	kilo	10^{3}	thousand
M	mega	10^{6}	million
G	giga	10^{9}	billion (thousand million)
T	tera	10^{12}	thousand billion
P	peta	10^{15}	million billion
E	exa	10^{18}	billion billion

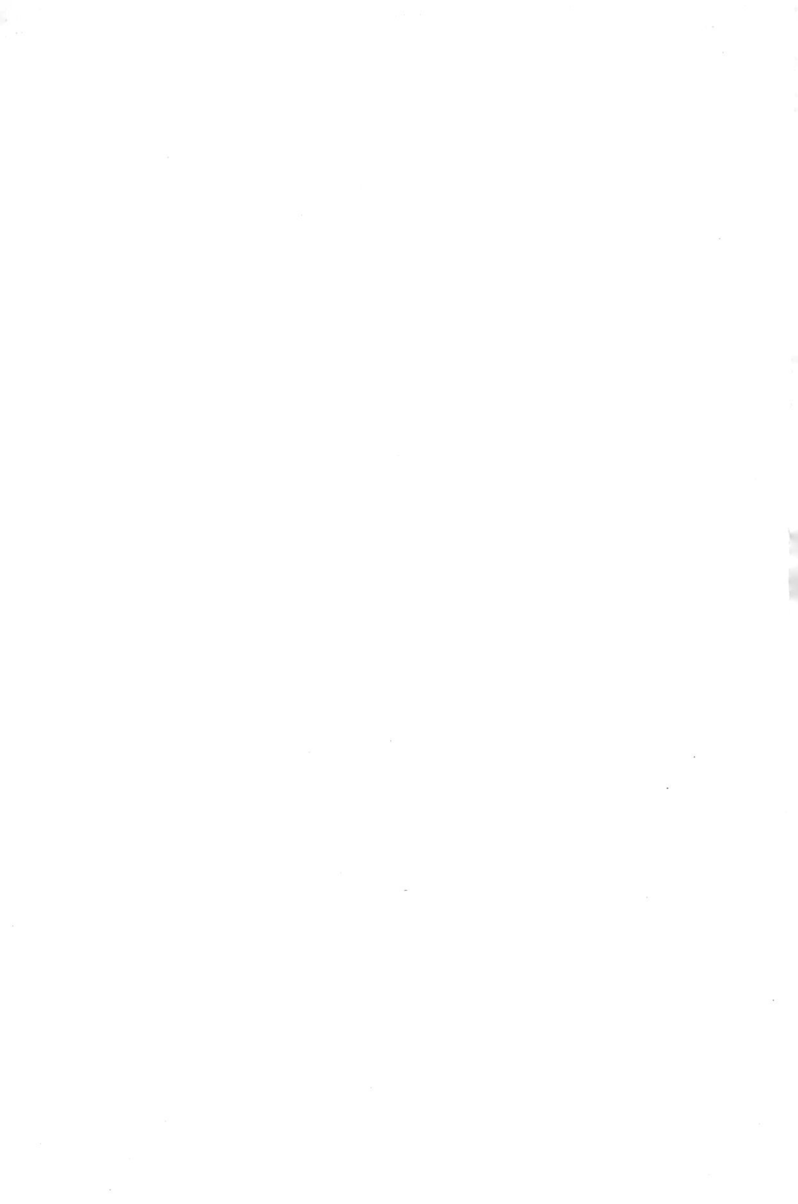